IMPORTANT INFORM

The information provided in this book is designed to provide helpful information on the subjects discussed. This book is not meant to be used, nor should it be used, to diagnose or treat any medical condition. For diagnosis or treatment of any medical problem, consult your own physician. The publisher and author are not responsible for any specific health or allergy needs that may require medical supervision and are not liable for any damages or negative consequences from any treatment, action, application or preparation, to any person reading or following the information in this book. References are provided for informational purposes only and do not constitute endorsement of any websites or other sources. Readers should be aware that the websites listed in this book may change.

WHAT THIS BOOK IS NOT!

Whilst I have referred where appropriate to important medically based studies, books and medical papers, this book has not been written as a medical research paper, designed to cover dozens of scientific subjects.

I have deliberately avoided the current trend in many diet books to constantly cherry pick medical and scientific studies to support the book's conclusions. This book is not intended as a reference item to satisfy those readers that might be looking for useful research material.

This book is about a real life journey and the real life testing processes that have identified the most effective ways to develop great eating behaviours and incorporating those behaviours into our daily food choices.

There will be a detailed bibliography attached to this book. This is a truly exciting and rapidly evolving science and there is a vast amount of material to read and study about Epigenetics, Ketogenics, Paleolithic Eating Selection and Functional Medicine in general, especially in the way that these insights apply to intelligent weight management. If you require further information, I suggest you contact me for specific recommendations at

beranparry@gmail.com

Copyright © 2015 by Beran Parry

All rights reserved. No part of this publication may be reproduced, distributed, or transmitted in any form or by any means, including photocopying, recording, or other electronic or mechanical methods, without the prior written permission of the publisher, except in the case of brief quotations embodied in critical reviews and certain other non-commercial uses permitted by copyright law. For permission requests, write to the author's email address: beranparry@gmail.com

Special Free Gift

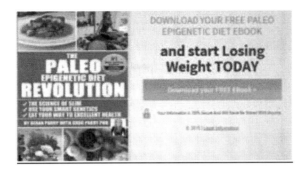

PLEASE VISIT OUR WEBSITES FREE BOOK PAGE to get your Free Gift

www.skinnydeliciouslife.com

BY THE SAME AUTHOR

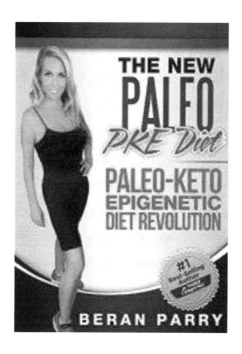

The New PKE DIET RECIPE BOOK

The UltimatePaleo-Keto-Epigenetic Blueprint

By

BERAN PARRY

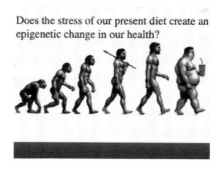

FROM THE AUTHOR

So much has changed in our understanding of how the human body functions. New research, dramatic developments in how we measure what happens inside our bodies, revolutionary shifts in the way we're applying this new knowledge to help people overcome serious medical conditions.

The Paleo movement resulted from a better understanding of how humans evolved and recognised that our bodies haven't changed fundamentally for tens of thousands of years. This led to a scientifically-endorsed approach to a more natural way of fuelling the body. The results have been astonishing, especially in terms of encouraging natural and sustained weight-loss and the relief of dozens of chronic medical problems.

One of the surprising conclusions from the Paleo research is that humans have not adapted successfully to large-scale grain consumption. We consume far too many carbohydrates and, as our bodies convert the carbs to glucose, we experience a range of inflammatory conditions as well major increases in weight.

The Keto Diet simply acknowledges how our ancestors fuelled their bodies for thousands of generations. The surprising answer that the Paleo and Keto Diets reveal is that a low-carb, moderate-protein and high-fat diet is natural the key to producing the ketones that burn our body fat as fuel, instead of converting carbs into energy. Most surprising is the fact that our muscles and organs - including our brains - prefer to function on ketones rather than on carb-based glucose. It's how we evolved. So, if you want to lose weight, one of the essential ingredients that's probably missing from your diet - is fat!

You might still hear the occasional explanation that bad genes account for so much excess weight, disease or ill-health. It's time to put that outdated and misleading concept in the rubbish bin where it belongs. This is where the most astonishing research into human genetics has demonstrated that many of our genes are not fixed. They can be switched on and off. That means that genetic indicators for many medical conditions can be influenced by environmental factors - and that includes the food we eat. That's right. We can no longer blame our ancestors for all of our inherited conditions. It's about lifestyle choices and putting the responsibility for our health, our weight and our wellbeing firmly back in our own hands. The PKE Dietary Revolution and Recipe Book listens to your body and helps you to feel as amazing as your body really wants you to feel. The Revolutionary begins today!

also

BY THE BEST SELLING AUTHOR

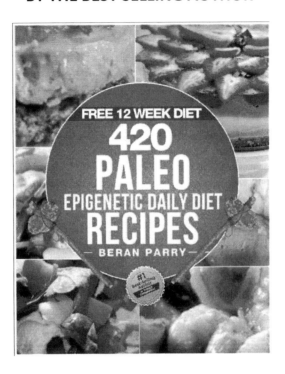

Table of Contents

Table of Contents

Preface

Chapter 1

My Story

Chapter 2

So Why Can't I Lose Weight? And why can't I keep the weight off?

Chapter 3

Epigenetics + PALEO/KETO Eating Behaviours

    The PALEO-KETO EPIGENETIC EATING PROGRAM – what is it?

Chapter 4

The Epigenetic Mythbuster Chart

Chapter5

Getting Organised to make Epigenetic Eating Behaviour more Effective!

Chapter 6

Epigenetic GUT BIOLOGY

Chapter 7

YOUR Paleo – Keto - Epigenetic Eating Transformation

Chapter 8

Toxins and genetic interference – causing weight loss problems

Chapter 9

Index to PKE Recipes

    BREAKFASTS – No Grain

    EGGIE MEALS

    MAIN COURSE - CHICKEN

    MAIN COURSE – FISH

    SALAD – ANIMAL PROTEIN

    PURE VEGETABLES – PLEASE ADD ANY RAW NUTS and/or AVOCADO TO OBTAIN THE KETO FAT REQUIREMENT ON ALL THESE RECIPES!

    DESERTS

    SMOOTHIES

    SNACKS

SOUPS

Chapter 10

The PKE DIET REVOLUTION Plan

   PALEO EPIGENETIC RECIPES

   PALEO EPIGENETIC RECIPES

Paleo Epigenetic Breakfasts (Grain Free)

1. Gutsy Granola
2. Spicy Granola
3. High Protein Breakfast Gold
4. Apple Breakfast Dream
5. Divine Protein Muesli
6. Ultimate Skinny Granola
7. Apple Chia Delight
8. Tasty Apple Almond Coconut Medley
9. Choco Nut Skinny Muesli Balls
10. Sweetie Skinny Crackers

Paleo Epigenetic Egg Meals

1. Scrambled Eggs with Chilli
2. Basil and Walnut Eggs Divine
3. Spicy Scrambled Eggs
4. Spicy India Omelet
5. Spectacular Spinach Omelet
6. Blushing Blueberry Omelet
7. Mediterranean Supercharger Omelet with Fennel and Dill
8. Outstanding Veggie Omelette
9. Spicy Spinach Bake
10. Delish Veggie Hash With Eggs
11. Spectacular Eggie Salsa
12. Mushrooms, Eggs and Onion Bonanza
13. Avocado and Shrimp Omelet
14. Delish Veggie Breakfast Peppers
15. Breakfast Mexicana

16. Zucchini Casserole
17. Blueberry Nut Casserole

Paleo Epigenetic Main Meals (Lunch or Dinner)

Paleo Epigenetic Poultry & Game

1. Spicy Turkey Stir Fry
2. Turkey and Kale Pasta Casserole
3. Roasted Lemon Herb Chicken
4. Basil Turkey with Roasted Tomatoes
5. Roasted and Filled Tasty Bell Peppers
6. Chili-Garlic Ostrich or Venison Skewers
7. Creamy Chicken Casserole
8. Spectacular Spaghetti and Delish Turkey Balls
9. Sensational Courgette Pasta and Turkey Bolognaise
10. Tempting Turkey Spaghetti Squash Boats
11. Delicious Turkey Veggie Lasagna
12. Ostrich Steak or Venison with Divine Mustard Sauce and Roasted Tomatoes
13. Tantalizing Turkey Pepper Stir-fry
14. Cheeky Chicken Stir Fry
15. Perfect Eastern Turkey Stir-Fry
16. Creamy Curry Stir Fry
17. Sexy Turkey Scramble
18. Turkey Thai Basil
19. Chicken Fennel Stir-Fry
20. Moroccan Madness

Paleo Epigenetic Fish

21. Thai Baked Fish with Squash Noodles
22. Divine Prawn Mexicana
23. Superior Salmon with Lemon and Thyme OR Use any White fish
24. Spectacular Shrimp Scampi in Spaghetti Sauce
25. Scrumptious Cod in Delish Sauce
26. Delish Baked dill Salmon
27. Prawn garlic Fried "Rice"

28. Lemon and Thyme Super Salmon
29. Delicious Salmon in Herb Crust
30. Salmon Mustard Delish
31. Sexy Spicy Salmon
32. Mouthwatering Stuffed Salmon
33. Spectacular Salmon
34. Creamy Coconut Salmon
35. Salmon Dill Bonanza
36. Sexy Shrimp Cocktail
37. Gambas al Ajillo--Sizzling Garlic Shrimp
38. Garlic Lemon Shrimp Bonanza
39. Courgette Pesto and Shrimp
40. Easy Shrimp Stir Fry
41. Delectable Shrimp Scampi
42. Citrus Shrimp Delux
43. Sexy Garlic Shrimp
44. Shrimp Cakes Delux
45. Shrimp Spinach Spectacular
46. Prawn Salad Boats
47. Cheeky Curry Shrimp
48. Courgette Shrimp Noodles
49. Sexy Shrimp on Sticks
50. Delicious Fish Stir Fry
51. Sexy Shrimp with Delish Veggie Stir Fry

Paleo Epigenetic Salads

1. Skinny Delicious Slaw
2. Turkey Eastern Surprise
3. Mediterranean Turkey Delish Salad
4. Skinny Delicious Turkey Divine
5. Chicken Basil Avo Salad
6. Skinny Chicken salad
7. Turkey Taco Salad

8. Cheeky Turkey Salad
9. Macadamia Chicken Salad
10. Rosy Chicken Supreme Salad
11. Turkey Sprouts Salad
12. Delicious Chicken Salad
13. Avocado Tuna Salad
14. Classic Tuna Salad
15. Artichoke Tuna Delight
16. Tasty Tuna Stuffed Tomato
17. Advanced Avocado Tuna Salad
18. Sexy Italian Tuna Salad
19. Divine Chicken or Turkey and Baby Bok Choy Salad
20. Mediterranean Medley Salad
21. Spicy Eastern Salad
22. Basil Avocado Bonanza Salad
23. Chinese Divine Salad
24. Divinely Delish Salad Surprise
25. Avocado Salad with Cilantro and Lime
26. Mexican Medley Salad
27. Macadamia Nut Chicken/Turkey Salad
28. Red Cabbage Bonanza Salad
29. Spectacular Sprouts Salad
30. Avocado Egg Salad
31. Avocado Divine Salad
32. Classic Waldorf Salad
33. Artichoke Heart & Turkey Salad Radicchio Cups
34. Tempting Tuna Stuffed Tomato
35. Incredibly Delish Avocado Tuna Salad
36. Italian Tuna Bonanza Salad
37. Asian Aspiration Salad
38. Tasty Carrot Salad
39. Creamy Carrot Salad

Paleo Epigenetic Pure Vegetables

1. Vegetarian Curry with Squash
2. Saucy Gratin with Creamy Cauliflower Bonanza
3. Egg Bok Choy and Basil Stir-Fry
4. Skinny Eggie Vegetable Stir Fry
5. Rucola Salad
6. Tasty Spring Salad
7. Spinach and Dandelion Pomegranate Salad
8. Pure Delish Spinach Salad
9. Sexy Salsa Salad
10. Eastern Avo Salad
11. Curry Coconut Salad
12. Jalapeno Salsa
13. Beet Sprout Divine Salad
14. Divine Carrot Salad
15. Cauliflower Couscous
16. Mouthwatering Mushroom Salad
17. Skinny Sweet Potato Salad

Paleo Epigenetic Desserts

1. Fabulous Brownie Treats
2. Rose Banana Delicious Brownies
3. Pristine Pumpkin Divine
4. Secret Brownies
5. Spectacular Spinach Brownies
6. Choco-coco Brownies
7. Coco – Walnut Brownie Bites
8. Best Ever Banana Surprise Cake
9. Choco Cookie Delight
10. Choco Triple Delight
11. Peach and Almond Cake
12. Apple Cinnamon Walnut Bonanza
13. Chestnut- Cacao Cake

14. Extra Dark Choco Delight
15. Nut Butter Truffles
16. Fetching Fudge
17. Choco – Almond Delights
18. Chococups
19. Choco Coco Cookies
20. Apple Spice Spectacular
21. Absolute Almond Bites
22. Eastern Spice Delights
23. Berry Ice Cream and Almond Delight
24. Creamy Caramely Ice Cream
25. Cheeky Cherry Ice
26. Choco - Coconut Berry Ice
27. Creamy Berrie Pie
28. Peachy Creamy Peaches
29. Spiced Apple Bake
30. Sexy Dessert Pan
31. Pretty Pumpkin Delights
32. Macadamia Pineapple Bonanza
33. Lemony Lemon Delights

Paleo Epigenetic Smoothies

1. Gorgeous Berry Smoothie
2. Tempting Coconut Berry Smoothie
3. Volumptious Vanilla Hot Drink
4. Almond Butter Smoothies
5. Choco Walnut Delight
6. Raspberry Hemp Smoothie
7. Choco Banana Smoothie
8. Blueberry Almond Smoothie
9. Hazelnut Butter and Banana Smoothie
10. Vanilla Blueberry Smoothie
11. Chocolate Raspberry Smoothie

12. Peach Smoothie
13. Zesty Citrus Smoothie
14. Apple Smoothie
15. Pineapple Smoothie
16. Strawberry Smoothie
17. Pineapple Coconut Deluxe Smoothie
18. Divine Vanilla Smoothie
19. Coco Orange Delish Smoothie
20. Baby Kale Pineapple Smoothie
21. Sumptuous Strawberry Coconut Smoothie
22. Blueberry Bonanza Smoothies
23. Divine Peach Coconut Smoothie
24. Tantalizing Key Lime Pie Smoothie
25. High Protein and Nutritional Delish Smoothie
26. Pineapple Protein Smoothie
27. Raspberry Coconut Smoothie
28. Ginger Carrot Protein Smoothie

Paleo Epigenetic Snacks

1. Delish Banana Nut Muffins
2. Delightful Cinnamon Apple Muffins
3. Healthy Breakfast Bonanza Muffins
4. Perfect Pumpkin Seeds
5. Gorgeous Spicy Nuts
6. Krunchy Yummy Kale Chips
7. Delicious Cinnamon Apple Chips
8. Gummy Citrus Snack
9. Skinny Veggie Dip
10. Divine Butternut Chips
11. Outstanding Orange Skinny Snack
12. Spicy Pumpkin Seed Bonanza
13. Delectable Chocolate-Frosted Doughnuts
14. Eggplant Divine

15. Choco Apple Nachos
16. Skinny Delicious Snack Bars
17. Pumpkin Vanilla Delight
18. Skinny Quicky Crackers
19. Delectable Parsnip Chips
20. Spicy Crunchy Skinny Snack
21. Raw Hemp Kale Bars
22. Skinny Trail Mix
23. Anti-Aging Fruit Delights
24. Paleo Rosemary Sweet Potato Crunches
25. Apple Peach Skinny Bars
26. Spicy Fried Almonds
27. Zucchini Avocado Hummus
28. Skinny Power Snack
29. Skinny Salsa
30. Divine Turkey Stuffed Tomatoes
31. Curried Nutty Delish
32. Skinny Chips
33. Zesty Zucchini Pesto Roll-ups
34. Butternut Squash-raw Veggie Dip
35. Skinny Power Balls
36. Chocolate Goji Skinny Bars
37. Delish Cashew Butter Treats

Paleo Epigenetic Soups

1. Roasted Tasty Tomato Soup
2. Thai Coconut Turkey Soup
3. Cheeky Chicken Soup
4. Triple Squash Delight Soup
5. Ginger Carrot Delight Soup
6. Wonderful Watercress Soup
7. Curried Butternut Soup
8. Celery Cashew Cream Soup

9. Mighty Andalusian Gazpacho
10. Munchy Mushroom Soup
11. Tempting Tomato Basil Soup
12. Healing Chicken/Turkey Vegetable Soup
13. Sumptuous Saffron Turkey Cauliflower Soup
14. Delicious Masala Soup
15. Creamy Chicken Soup
16. Delicious Lemon-Garlic Soup
17. Turkey Squash Soup
18. Roasted Winter Vegetable Turkey Soup
19. Zucchini Fish Soup Delight!

Chapter 11

The PKE Vision

About the Author

Bibliography

FREE BONUS CHAPTER

Preface

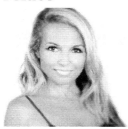

The Amazing PALEO-KETOEpigenetic Eating Program and Recipe Book did not appear magically overnight or out of thin air. It's the result of many years of research, trial, tribulation and intensive investigation.

As an internationally recognised nutrition and wellbeing specialist who consults around the world, I advise clients on the best eating strategies for health and weight control.

I develop nutritional and exercise programs, analyse eating behaviour and I have designed effective weight loss strategies for thousands of international clients.

I am committed to helping you find your ideal wellbeing using dynamic weight control strategies like Paleo, Keto, Vegan and Functional Medicine Diagnostics.

I have studied nutritional therapy, passing over 10 exams.. as well as obtaining certification in eating disorders, hormone balance and sports nutrition, as well as hands on experience in ayurvedic nutrition.

Despite studying nutrition intensively for over 30 years, I found that I never really reached the permanent weight loss that I wanted. No matter how much weight I lost, I was never really where I wanted to be with my weight.

That has got to be one of the greatest frustrations you can experience when you're trying to get your weight under control. There was usually some initial success but then there'd be some unexpected relapse and this made me realise that there had to be a lot more to real, sustainable weight loss than just following the latest fad or fashion in dieting.

But I never gave up.

If permanent weight loss and becoming a leaner, healthier version of myself was really possible, I was going to find out how to do it. Safely, scientifically and effectively. And that meant more studying, more learning, more experiments, more trials, more creativity, inventing, developing. I approached the problem from every possible angle.

I researched countless scientific studies, the psychological aspects of food choice, the psychology of eating disorders, genetic analysis, functional medicine, naturopathic principles and ayurvedic medicine until a clear picture finally emerged of how to really manage weight issues.

I slowly refined and toned and developed the entire system that has become the Paleo-Keto - Epigenetic Eating Program. It's what you're holding in your hands right now. It's been a long journey but the effort was totally worthwhile. Finally, we've got the smart way for your body to function the way that Nature intended.

The PKE Diet represents one of the most advanced approaches to sustainable wright-loss in the world today and the recipes that have been prepared for you are as much a reward for your change in eating habits as a tool to improve your health beyond your wildest expectations. The recipes are purposefully aimed at being delicious. You really can enjoy your new, life-changing diet and take real pleasure from every bite in every meal. Life, after all, is a gift to be enjoyed and great-tasting food is something we can all appreciate. But beyond the mouth-watering varieties of super-nutrients contained in these super-advanced recipes, there is the knowledge and certainty that you are turning your life in a new direction, that you are following a pathway to amazing, natural weight-loss and that your health and wellbeing are receiving the help, support and encouragement that they truly deserve. Enjoy these fabulous recipes. You've made a fabulous choice with the PKE Diet. You absolutely deserve to enjoy all the rewards and benefits.

The Paleo-Keto Epigenetic Eating methods have already helped countless numbers of people just like you who were looking for a real alternative to all the crazy ideas about weight management.

The Paleo-Keto Epigenetic Eating process enables me to look you in the eye and say I KNOW this WORKS. And now you can enjoy the benefits yourself.

The Paleo-Keto-Epigenetic Recipe Book delivers deliciously tastes, mouth-watering menus and weight-loss cooking at its best! Enjoy your food and lose weight!

Whatever your age, your weight, your gender, the state of your hormones, your current adopted eating behaviour, we are going to work together to make your potential intelligent eating habits into your smart permanent eating behaviour by supplying you with over 250 recipes so that you can become your best body weight and realise your own potential for your best body shape ever!. And keep it forever!

Let's Start

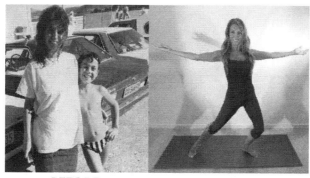

BEFORE　　　　　　　AFTER

Chapter 1

My Story

Welcome to the start of a whole new way of life! We're about to embark on an adventure together and my job is to help and guide you on your new pathway to the health, weight and wellbeing of your dreams. My name is Beran Parry and for the past thirty-five years I've been studying, practising and advising thousands of people about truly effective nutrition and weight loss. A lot of this passion comes from my family background. Growing up in a family with major health and weight problems, I realised at a very early age that body shape, weight and health are all deeply connected. To complicate matters, I became pregnant at the tender age of 18 and I experienced all the dismay and daily disappointment of significant weight gain plus the frustration of struggling to get rid of the extra pounds after giving birth to my lovely son Christopher.

By the time I was twenty-two, more than thirty years ago, I began studying nutrition, exercise physiology, integrative medicine and holistic health. I was immensely fortunate to find myself studying at one of the early pioneering centres of Integrative Alternative Medicine. This was the world renowned High Rustenberg Hydro, set in the beautiful countryside around Stellenbosch University, not far from my birthplace, Cape Town, in South Africa.

I studied very intensively for four years under the guidance of various medical and homeopathic doctors whilst also studying banking and finance. My studies continued right up until 1986 when I moved from South Africa to Europe.

The most exciting news to emerge from the latest scientific research on human metabolism is that we really can choose how our bodies look and behave. It's really a question of controlling the influences that determine how our bodies function and right at top of that list of influences is the way we eat. We're entering a revolutionary phase in our understanding of how the human body functions, letting go of outdated concepts and myths and balancing our health needs with the most up to date revelations about human physiology.

The conclusions from all of this pioneering and often surprising research is that our bodies function best on a low-carb, medium-protein and relatively high-fat dietary regime. We certainly didn't evolve to live off the grain-rich foods that form the basis of the western diet.

Grains are largely inflammatory and encourage the storage of fat, two particular problems that are damaging the health of hundreds of millions of people around the world every day. The old advice to cut down on fats has produced a completely unexpected rise in obesity rates and many medical practitioners have been confused and frustrated by the results of their well-meant advice to patients to cut fat out of their diets. The rise in obesity rates continues. So we understand now that humans need fat in their diets in order to metabolise the fat that's been stored in their bodies. We also recognise today that cutting out grains and sugars can have a powerful and dramatic impact on health and weight-loss issues.

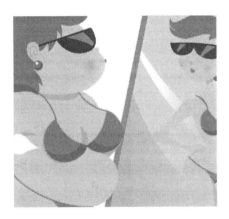

Chapter 2

So Why Can't I Lose Weight? And why can't I keep the weight off?

These are good questions because even champion weight losers often put the weight back on, suffering the seemingly inevitable see-saw effect of cyclical weight loss followed by weight gain. Can we do something to correct this problem? Of course we can! That's exactly what this book is for.

Epigenetic PARADIGM PYRAMID 1 – YOUR BIGGEST WEIGHT INFLUENCER

YOUR Inherited GENETICS - 10%

Genes can be outsmarted by epigenetics

Your Gut holds the Secrets of Healthy Weightloss

YOUR FOOD SELECTION PROCESS – 30%

What and When YOU Eat Makes the Difference

Your Food Choices are the Critical Factor

Your Challenge is to really Learn how to Eat Smart, Eat Right and Feel Great

YOUR Epigenetic Eating BEHAVIOUR and Epigenetic Expression 60%

Eating Behaviour Rules the Scales

Personal Choices Always Produce Inevitable Consequences

Choosing the Right Priorities when it comes to What and How and When we Eat,

Time Management when it relates to your Eating Behaviour can be your biggest Friend or Enemy

If you would like to learn more about the New Paleo PKE Diet, we suggest you download the initial book in this series

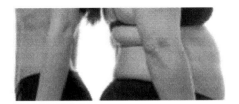

Chapter 3

Epigenetics + PALEO/KETO Eating Behaviours

Epi – WHAT??

Perhaps you haven't heard all the excitement in medical and scientific circles about the latest revelations in the field of Epigenetics. Epi-what? OK. Before we go any further, you're probably wondering what on earth Epigenetics really means. Is it contagious? Can we get it at the grocery store? Does it come in my size? So let's start by answering an important question: "What exactly is Epigenetics?"

The formal description of Epigenetics from the text books refers to the study of changes in organisms caused by modification of gene expression rather than by an alteration of the genetic code itself. That might not tell us very much but it really is an important statement! It's no longer simply a case of identifying which particular genes you have.

We now know that it's the way your genes are influenced and made to work that makes the difference. Gene expression accounts for so many of our characteristics. And changes in gene expression have been related to a very wide range of environmental influences and that includes – are you ready for this? – What we eat!

Yes, that's absolutely right. The kind of food we consume every single day, the quality of the food we eat, the eating choices we make all contribute far more to our total health and wellbeing than was ever appreciated before. It's not a question of being pre-programmed by our DNA. We've been bombarded by articles and news items for decades telling us every day that everything in our lives is caused by our genes.

The PALEO-KETO EPIGENETIC EATING PROGRAM – what is it?

The PALEO-KETO Epigenetic Eating Three Golden Food Rules!

1. Weight loss is all about insulin

Moderate your insulin production levels by eliminating sugar and grains (yes, even whole grains) and you will lose the excess body fat without dieting - plus you will improve your energy levels, reduce inflammation throughout the body and eliminate disease risk. Maybe this should be printed in a very large font size in the brightest colour your printer can produce!

2. Eating lean…… protein but plenty good quality fat

Vegetable and some correctly sourced animal protein with high good fat content is not only healthy but is the key to effortless weight loss, a healthy immune system and boundless energy.

3. Eat Clean

When we examine the role that food plays in avoiding or encouraging weight gain, you might be shocked to discover that one of the biggest influences is concealed in the way that our food is processed. Hold onto your hat, my friend. This can get scary! The most significant components of food that play the largest role in weight gain and obesity are food additives, chemicals, and food processing techniques.

It's time to get some much needed clarity into the discussion. So, let's begin by asking – What exactly is the Ketogenic Diet?

KETOGENICS

We're going to start by defining precisely what ketosis is and why it's so important for so many aspects of our health and wellbeing, and that includes sustainable weight loss too.

Ketosis (pronounced KEY-TOE-SIS) is a word that describes the metabolic state that occurs when you consume a very low-carb, moderate-protein, high-fat diet. Ketosis causes your body to switch from using glucose as its primary source of fuel to running on ketones. Ketones themselves are produced when the body burns fat, and they're primarily used as an alternative fuel source when glucose isn't available.

In other words, in the simplest and most dramatic way of summing up the process, your body changes from a sugar-burner to a fat-burner. Depending on your current diet and lifestyle choices, becoming keto-adapted can take as little as a few days and or as much as several weeks. In some cases it's even taken months. So "being in ketosis" just means that you are burning fat. You might need some good, old-fashioned, patience and persistence but the range of benefits absolutely justifies the effort as you pursue ketosis.

Here are some of the many health benefits that come from being in ketosis: (DISCLAIMER – Some of these benefits may be hampered by poor health and lifestyle choices in other areas than diet!)

- Natural hunger and appetite control
- Effortless weight loss and maintenance
- Mental clarity
- Sounder, more restful sleep
- Normalized metabolic function
- Stabilized blood sugar and restored insulin sensitivity
- Lower inflammation levels
- Feelings of happiness and general well-being

- Lowered blood pressure
- Increased HDL (good) cholesterol
- Reduced triglycerides
- Lowered or eliminated small LDL particles (bad cholesterol)
- Ability to go twelve to twenty-four hours between meals
- Use of stored body fat as a fuel source
- Endless energy
- Eliminated heartburn
- Better fertility
- Prevention of traumatic brain injury
- Increased sex drive
- Improved immune system
- Slowed aging due to reduction in free radical production
- Improvements in blood chemistry
- Optimized cognitive function and improved memory
- Reduced acne breakouts and other skin conditions
- Heightened understanding of how foods affect your body
- Improvements in metabolic health markers
- Faster and better recovery from exercise
- Decreased anxiety and mood swings

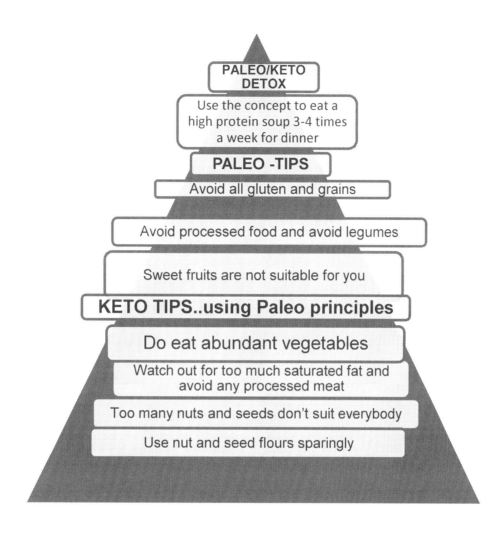

If you would like to learn more about the New Paleo PKE Diet, we suggest you download the initial book in this series

Summary - Epigenetics

Your genetic profile is not the full story

Your genes can be switched on and off

The food you eat is the key to influencing your genetic responses

Methylation and diet change the rules of the genetic game

Managing insulin levels by eliminating all grains

Eat Lean, Clean and Good fats

Take practical steps to address food addiction

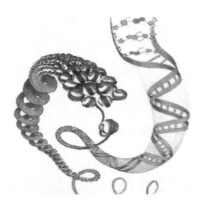

Chapter 4

The Epigenetic Mythbuster Chart

The Epigenetic Mythbuster Chart.....your 5 point blueprint and lifelong passport to the happy realm of total weight control and permanent residence in the Land of Leaner.

CMR Conventional Medical Recommendation.

DEFINITION: The old view of what is supposed to be good for you.

EPS Epigenetic Paradigm Shift.

DEFINITION: The revolutionary new advances in medical and scientific research that will transform your health

Let's get serious. Fact: If the old ways worked, we wouldn't be having an explosion of obesity in the developed world and we wouldn't be having this conversation, would we? Clearly something is missing. Our mission is to show you what the problem really is, how to fix the problem and fix it forever.

Step 1: Grains

>   **CMR:** Insists that grains are actually good for you. Wheat, rice, corn, cereal, bread, pasta etc. Most governments recommend 8-10 servings per day as the principle daily source of energy, nutrition and fiber. Entire industries are devoted to promoting

this idea as the healthiest way to live. Ask pretty much anyone and they'll tell you how good it is to eat grains.

EPS: UCLA lecturer and world famous evolutionary biologist Jared Diamond stipulates "Grains are the worst mistake of the human race." In nutritional terms, grains are simply inferior to plants. Grains trigger insulin production and fat storage.

They produce allergic reactions, suppress the immune response and trigger a wide range of intolerances as well as imbalances in the intestinal flora.

Step 2: Fats

CMR: Fat makes you fat therefore if you reduce fat you'll lose fat. The world is awash with countless 'fat free' and 'low fat' products and we have a ballooning obesity problem.

EPS: Good quality fat drives efficient fat and protein metabolism, encouraging weight loss and boosting energy levels.

Step 3: Meal Habits

CMR: Three square meals a day plus snacks are best to stave off hunger pangs and stabilize metabolism

EPS: Any steps to normalize your insulin production encourages your skinny genes to take over. Occasional fasting using protein soup meals can help you to reprogram your fat burning potential

Step 4: Cardio exercise

CMR: 30-60 minutes cardio per day. Lift weights regularly using isolated parts of the body and aim for maximum resistance, even going for the point of failure to increase strength.

EPS: Weight resistance using the whole body in short bursts plus slower more regular cardio exercise for shorter periods per day with sporadic intense bursts of intensity. This system really does work!

Step 5: Sun exposure

CMR: Wear sunscreen every day, in all weather and in every season. It should have a sun protection factor (SPF) of 30 and say "broad-spectrum" on the label, which means it protects against the sun's UVA and UVB rays. Put it on at least 15 minutes before going outside. Use 1 ounce, which would fill a shot glass

EPS: Sunshine can be a tricky thing. We need it, but it can also be harmful.

Striking the right balance between getting enough sunshine to produce optimal levels of Vitamin D, and protecting ourselves from the harm the sun can do, can be a challenge. Most experts recommend 15-20 minutes of sun exposure several times a week for the average fair-skinned person, as this is enough to produce optimal levels of Vitamin D while not being so much to damage skin. Darker skin tones with more melanin need to stay in the sun longer to synthesize vitamin D effectively...see more info below

Vitamin D, which our body produces when we are exposed to sunlight, does wonders for us – from improving mood to boosting our immune systems, reducing inflammation and much more, it's key to our health.

According to some new research, it seems there is yet another reason to get the right amount of sunlight. Researchers found that older women (65+) with low Vitamin D levels are more likely to gain weight.

If you would like to learn more about the New Paleo PKE Diet, we suggest you download the initial book in this series

Summary - Mythbuster

The folly of grains in the human diet

Welcome to the inner universe of your microbiome

Being overweight is closely connected to the state of your gut flora

CMR versus EPS (epigenetic paradigm shift)

EPS - The smarter way to live long, lose weight and live better

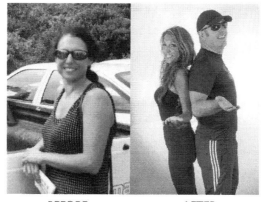

BEFORE   AFTER

Chapter 5

Getting Organised to make Epigenetic Eating Behaviour more Effective!

5 Steps to Re Organising Your Permanent Weight Reduction and Leaner Pathway!

Time to re-programme your food choices and eating behaviour

We are going to learn how to:

Exorcise the past and be free of old habits

Why we prioritise our activities in the wrong order

I've heard it so often, it's almost become the mantra of the unwilling, the permanent excuse for letting things slide. "There just isn't enough time to eat healthily and plan special meals, let alone shop or cook them or take them with me when I'm out of the house."

Sound familiar? ...here are more excuses.....

I feel so awful when I've eaten badly.

I feel such a failure.

My life is a mess.

Why is it such a struggle to lose weight?"

The result is a fairly miserable outlook and a lack of confidence, an unwillingness to recognise what is possible. The mind-set of the victim. But we're here to address these issues. We want you to feel the confidence that comes from daily, planned success. And getting organised takes all the pain and doubt from the process.

The irony is that the people who claim there's no time to incorporate these important changes in their lives have often been completely successful in other areas of their lives. Their success shows up in an infinite number of ways: they were incredibly accomplished managers or employees, highly creative artistic individuals, massively good parents or even someone who was good at something else. Every time you make a decision to do something, you're engaging your creative power. All we have to do is harness that potential.

Unhappiness can undoubtedly play its part in the way we treat our bodies. If you have doubts about your self-worth - I know, welcome to the human condition! - It often shows up in unhealthy eating habits and poor choices. It's a huge area and so important that it will be the subject of a future book.

That's why I'd like to encourage you to do something incredibly powerful right now. I want you to look in the mirror for a few moments. And smile. That's right. Smile. Look at yourself and smile. Your conscious mind might feel that the act is a little silly but your subconscious - and your body - will begin to get the message that you're giving them your personal stamp of approval. Have you ever noticed how a small child lights up when you really smile at them? Your body needs exactly that same recognition, that same high wattage smile of approval. Do it every time you step into the bathroom. Look into the mirror and smile. The results will amaze you.

We want your body and your subconscious to work with you. Give them that dazzling smile and you will find your body begins to co-operate in the most extraordinary ways. Try it. It's a very powerful technique for removing behavioural obstacles and we want to make this entire process as easy and comfortable as possible.

This entire book is designed to help you take control of your health, your weight and ultimately your happiness. Being kind to yourself, respecting the miracle of your body, learning to enjoy living in such an extraordinary structure, optimising its potential and being at peace with yourself. These are powerful keys to a very fulfilling way of experiencing the gift of life.

So the underlying theme to these methods is to be kind to yourself. To do things that benefit rather than harm your health. To respect your body's needs and live life to the full.

An abiding love and acceptance of yourself, despite all the imperfections, really helps you to overcome any harmful habits and behaviours and puts an end to the self-criticism and self-loathing that lowers self esteem and sabotages our efforts. It really is extraordinary how quickly we can change our lives simply by learning to accept ourselves and focus not on what might be amiss but on how we truly want to be.

If you would like to learn more about eating behaviour and the New Paleo PKE Diet, we suggest you download the initial book in this series

1. Identify your behaviours and habits.

I suggest taking a look at my Emotional Eating Book to further assist you in this area

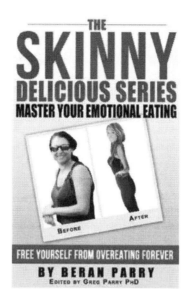

2. TAKE THE EATING BEHAVIOUR TEST

Follow this link to take the test

http://www.skinnydeliciouslife.com

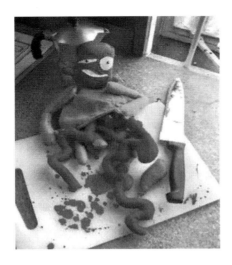

https://www.flickr.com/photos/tombland/51524073

Chapter 6

Epigenetic GUT BIOLOGY

Your gut biology and the secrets of effective, sustained weight loss

Let's get right down to the guts of the matter! Whilst countless diet books have focused on fads and fleeting feeding fashions, we've had to wait until now to discover that the key to successful weight control is hidden in our intestinal flora. Encouraging the right balance of microbes in our gut and enhancing natural digestion are two of the most important and positive contributions we can make towards generating great health and real weight control.

There is an ancient tradition in many cultures that our intelligence is not simply located in the brain. You might find it surprising that recent research is taking a fresh look at this unusual question and producing some unexpected answers.

Dr Natasha Campbell McBride, an authority in this fascinating area, states "The importance of your gut flora, and its influence on your health cannot be overstated. It is truly profound. Your gut literally serves as your second brain and even produces more of the neurotransmitter serotonin - known to have a beneficial influence on your mood - than your brain does".

It gets better.

If you would like to learn more about the New Paleo PKE Diet, we suggest you download the initial book in this series

Gut Biology Summary

The gut is the site of the 'second brain'

Inflammatory conditions are deeply influenced by the microbiome

Correcting intestinal flora is the key to health and weight loss

Identify the toxins that harm the body and disrupt normal gut functioning

Eliminate harmful substances from daily diet to restore balance

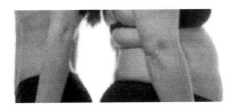

Chapter 7

YOUR Paleo – Keto - Epigenetic Eating Transformation

Welcome to Your brand new and exciting career! You are now Managing Director of Your Paleo-Keto Epigenetic Eating Life. Inc. Congratulations. It's simply the Best Job in the Whole World and now it's yours.

Your most important job from now on is to focus on making the right food choices. You don't need to weigh or measure, you don't need to count calories. Wow, I bet that sounds like a new way of dealing with the old weight loss issue, doesn't it? Just make that one decision to follow the programme under any and all circumstances, under any amount of stress and your body will do the rest.

Your only job?

The most important job in your life!

Eat The Right Food for Your Epigenetic Expression

Fall madly in love with your absolute best weight-loss foods - and watch them fall in love with you and your new, leaner body

From all the information you've absorbed so far, you'll know for sure that certain food groups (like sugars, grains and dairy products) could be having a very negative impact on your health and wellbeing without you even noticing. But when you think about your present state of wellbeing, you might be wondering how much of your health - or lack of it - has been caused by the food you've been eating. Weight loss is a great example. If you've tried to lose weight but always found it a struggle, experiencing initial success but then putting the pounds back on, you know that you have to do something different. It's time to recognise that cutting down the calories isn't enough. If you're still eating the wrong foods, the problems will remain. It's time to remove the source of the problem and that's only going to happen by removing all the harmful, toxic foods from your diet.

Say goodbye to all the psychologically unhealthy, hormone-unbalancing, gut-disrupting, inflammatory food groups and see the weight fall off. That's right. You might want to read that sentence again. It's essential to your future health. Let your body heal and recover from the years and years of weight gain and from all the other nasty effects of those nasty, toxic foods. It's time to re-programme your metabolism and flush away the inflammation.

Learn once and for all how the foods you've been eating are really affecting your health, your weight and your long term health. We've arrived at one of the most important reasons for you to follow this programme.

This is about to change your life.

Epigenetics demonstrates the vital link between the things you do and how you live to the way your body behaves, all the way down to the cellular level. This might be one of the most surprising revelations about the entire body transformation programme. I think you're going to like it because you're going to love the results.

We cannot possibly put enough emphasis on this simple fact.

Like many of the most important elements in our lives, the answers are so simple that it's too easy to blink and miss the power of this revelation.

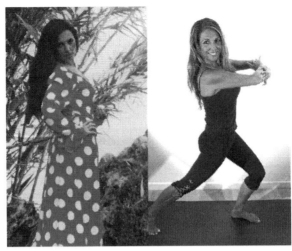

BEFORE　　　　AFTER

The Epigenetic Eating Transformation

Are you ready for this?

Well, take a deep breath, my friend, because this is the answer you've been waiting for.

Eat. Real. Food.

Eat real food.

Only eat real food.

And now you know.

Real food is unprocessed, additive free and as natural as nature intended.

Real food includes lean, organic game and poultry, line caught seafood, organic free range eggs, tons of fresh vegetables, some fruit, and plenty of good fats from fruits, oils, nuts and seeds.

Eat foods with very few ingredients and no additives, chemicals, sugars or flavourings. Better yet, eat foods with no ingredients listed at all because then they're totally natural and unprocessed.

Don't worry, these guidelines are outlined in extensive detail in our essential life-enhancing Epigenetic Eating Shopping list.

What to avoid if you want to be healthier, leaner and in better shape forever.

More importantly, here's what NOT to eat. Cutting out all of these foods and drinks will help you regain your natural, healthy metabolism, reduce systemic inflammation and help you to realise exactly how these foods are truly affecting your weight, fat percentage, health, fitness and every aspect of your life.

- Sugar. It's out. It's that simple. Do not consume added sugar of any kind whether it's real or artificial. No maple syrup, honey, agave nectar, coconut sugar, Splenda, Equal, Nutrasweet, Xylitol. The only exception is Stevia, the natural sweetener that avoids the toxicity of all the other sweeteners. Start reading the labels because food companies love to use sugar in their products to cater for your sugar addiction and they use it in ways you might not recognise. Great way to sell more products. Disastrous for your health.
- Do not consume beer in any form, not even for cooking. And let's be brutal about that other global addiction - tobacco. Absolutely no tobacco products of any sort. Ever. Wine though, in moderation, is fine. Ideally you'll opt for dry wines and a small amount of spirits but NO liqueurs ever!
- Do not eat grains. This includes wheat, rye, barley, oats, corn, rice, millet, bulgur, or sprouted grains
- The very occasional exceptions are buckwheat and quinoa which are not technically grains but, unfortunately, they have many grain like qualities. The answer is to limit your consumption and always exercise moderation. Cutting out grains also includes all the ways we add wheat, corn, rice and other starches to our foods in the form of bran, wheat germ, modified starch and so on. Again, read the labels.
- Do not eat legumes, except for some occasional sprouted legumes. This includes beans of all kinds (black, red, pinto, navy, white, kidney, lima, fava, etc.), peas, chickpeas, lentils, and peanuts. No peanut butter, either. This also includes all forms of soy, soy sauce, miso, tofu, tempeh, edamame and all the many ways we sneak soy into foods (like lecithin).
- Do not eat dairy. This includes cow, goat or sheep's milk and milk products such as cream, cheese (hard or soft), kefir, yogurt (even Greek), and sour cream. Use coconut milk, coconut yoghurt and coconut cream.
- Do not consume carrageenan, MSG, sulphites or any additives whatsoever. If these ingredients or any E numbers appear in any form on the label of your processed food or beverage, don't even touch it!.

Sounds tough, doesn't it? But that's because we've been conditioned to connect really bad food and sugary sweet flavourings with good times. We get sweets and candy as a reward during childhood and the comforting feeling gets embedded in our behaviour.

Before long we're addicted to all the things that effectively poison us. Take a look around you. Do you see much evidence of happy, healthy people in the local population? Disease incidence and obesity are ballooning. Something's radically wrong and you are one of the few, lucky ones to know exactly where the problem really lies.

Knowledge is power, my friend. Let's put this life-changing knowledge to the best possible use. Right now. You know what to do. All you have to do is make one powerful choice for health, normal weight and a tremendous increase in energy and the quality of your life and your body will do the rest.

At this stage of the programme, you might be surprised to know that we're not going to obsess too much about the weighting scales. The really important changes are taking place inside your body and your weight will improve naturally as you allow it to flush out all the toxins and reduce inflammation levels.

The Fine Print

The PALEO/KETO Epigenetic Shopping Guide

Being overweight is expensive in every possible way. And it costs far too much in terms of your quality of life. So it's vitally important to make healthy eating your absolute top priority and there are many of ways for you to maximize your food budget. We'll start with the top foods in the PALEO/KETO Epigenetic Eating Diet

The next three items ALL SHARE EQUAL PRIORITY

#1: Protein

Always start at the game, poultry, fish, and eggs section first because the majority of your budget should be spent on high quality animal protein.

- If you are against consuming animal protein for any reason, you have a great alternative in Hemp Protein Powder

Hemp protein, made from the hemp seed, is a high-fibre protein supplement that can be used to enhance total protein intake for vegans and non-vegans alike. Hemp can be considered a superior protein source due to its above-average digestibility, which also makes it ideal for athletes. When a protein is efficiently digested, it can be deployed more effectively by the body. The digestibility of any given protein is related to the concentrations of its amino acids. A study published in 2010 in the "Journal of Agricultural and Food Chemistry" tested the protein digestibility-corrected amino acid score (PDAAS) -- a rating that determines the bioavailability of a protein -- for various proteins derived from the hemp seed. The results showed that hemp seed proteins have PDAAS values greater than or equal to a variety of grains, nuts and legumes. We're big fans of hemp seed protein because it enhances the immune system and boosts energy levels as well as protecting the kidneys.

#2: Vegetables

Now that you've organised your essential protein supplies, it's time to move on to the vegetables. These are the second tier of your super new plan for effective weight loss and new levels of wellbeing.

- during the three week detox phase….after that always eat sparingly.
-

#3: Healthy Fats

Healthy fats make up the last but most important item on your shopping list. Some of the healthiest fats are also the least expensive and it's always a good idea to keep a good supply of oils, nuts, and seeds at home to help in preparing your super, new Epigenetic meals.

For a Full Detailed Shopping Guide – click through to our PKE Shopping List and Additional Items

www.skinnydeliciouslife.com

look for the free lists in the menu

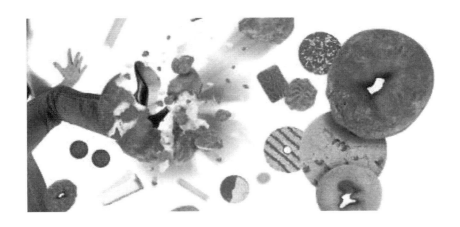

Chapter 8

Toxins and genetic interference – causing weight loss problems

Food processing or food poisoning techniques?

The modern industrial approach to food production and processing is responsible for a ghastly range of chemicals and additives that are directly involved in producing weight gain, fat and obesity. Amongst the thousands of additives, we have bovine growth hormone and antibiotics injected into meat, poultry, and dairy products, flavour enhancers such as monosodium glutamate, artificial sweeteners such as NutraSweet (aspartame) and Splenda (sucralose). Our list also includes man-made sugars such as high fructose corn syrup, corn syrup, dextrose, sucrose, fructose, highly refined white sugar, processed molasses, processed honey, maltodextrin, etc., plus the other 15,000 plus chemicals that are routinely added to virtually every product you buy, and that includes conventionally grown fruits and vegetables.

Man-made trans-fats such as hydrogenated or partially hydrogenated oils also cause weight gain and obesity. Even standard food processing techniques such as pasteurisation, which now applies to virtually every product in a bottle or carton, homogenisation and irradiation all contribute to weight gain.

At the end of this disturbing list of toxins, poisons and health-damaging additives we have some refreshing and deeply reassuring news. Your revolutionary epigenetic weight control system addresses all of these issues safely and effectively and offers the fast lane out of the nightmare of processed food. Once you know you have the tools to make things better, you can breathe a sigh of relief and start to take action..

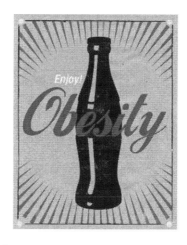

https://www.flickr.com/photos/melliegrunt/4457372401

OBESITY AND TOXICITY: What is the real connection?

Effects on Thyroid and Metabolic Rate

If you've ever attempted a weight loss programme, you'll probably recognise the familiar plateau phase where many people lose a few pounds but then find it really difficult to shed the rest.

What might be getting in the way of further weight loss and even interfering with the metabolic control system? A review paper, "Energy balance and pollution by organochlorines and polychlorinated biphenyls," published in Obesity Reviews in 2003 describes the effects of toxins on metabolic rate and weight regulation.

The authors conclude that pesticides (organochlorines) and PCBs (from industrial pollution), which are normally stored in fat tissue, are released during the weight loss process and lower the metabolic rate. That will slow down the rate at which we can lose the pounds. How do the chemical toxins interfere with our metabolism?

People with a higher body mass index (BMI) have a larger volume of places to hold onto the toxins. They store more toxins because they have more fat. Those toxins interfere with many normal aspects of metabolism, including reducing thyroid hormone levels, and increasing excretion of thyroid hormones via the liver.

If you would like to learn more about the New Paleo PKE Diet, we suggest you download the initial book in this series

Toxins Summary

Pollutions and toxins are everywhere

Obesity and toxicity are closely related

The power of leptins

The thyroid connection

Cleansing and healing the body for permanent weight control

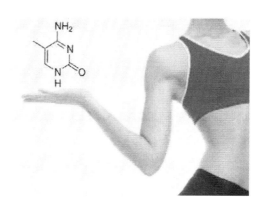

Chapter 9

Index to PKE Recipes

BREAKFASTS – No Grain
1. Gutsy Granola
2. Spicy Granola
3. High Protein Breakfast Gold
4. Apple Breakfast Dream
5. Divine Protein Muesli
6. Ultimate Skinny Granola
7. Apple Chia Delight
8. Tasty Apple Almond Coconut Medley
9. Choco Nut Skinny Muesli Balls
10. Sweetie Skinny Crackers

EGGIE MEALS
11. Scrambled Eggs with Chilli
12. Basil and Walnut Eggs Divine
13. Spicy Scrambled Eggs
14. Spicy India Omelette
15. Spectacular Spinach Omelette

16   Blushing Blueberry Omelette

17   Mediterranean Supercharger Omelette with Fennel and Dill

18   Outstanding Veggie Omelette

19   Spicy Spinach Bake

20   Delish Veggie Hash With Eggs

21   Spectacular Eggie Salsa

22   Mushrooms, Eggs and Onion Bonanza

23   Avocado and Shrimp Omelette

24   Delish Veggie Breakfast Peppers

25   Breakfast Mexicana

26   Zucchini Casserole

27   Blueberry Nut Casserole

MAIN COURSE - CHICKEN

28   Spicy Turkey Stir Fry

29   Turkey and Kale Pasta Casserole

30   Roasted Lemon Herb Chicken

31   Basil Turkey with Roasted Tomatoes

32   Roasted and Filled Tasty Bell Peppers

33   Chili-Garlic Ostrich or Venison Skewers

34   Creamy Chicken Casserole

35   Spectacular Spaghetti and delish turkey balls

36   Sensational Courgette Pasta and Turkey bolognaise

37   Tempting Turkey Spaghetti Squash Boats

38   Delicious Turkey Veggie Lasagna

39   Ostrich Steak or Venison with Divine Mustard Sauce and Roasted Tomatoes

40   Tantalizing Turkey Pepper Stir-fry

41	Cheeky Chicken Stir Fry
42	Perfect Turkey Stir-Fry
43	Creamy Curry Stir Fry
44	Sexy Turkey Scramble
45	Turkey Thai Basil
46	Chicken Fennel Stir-Fry
47	Moroccan Madness

MAIN COURSE – FISH

48	Thai Baked Fish with Squash Noodles
49	Divine Prawn Mexicana
50	Superior Salmon with Lemon and Thyme – OR - Use any White fish
51	Spectacular Shrimp Scampi in spaghetti sauce
52	Scrumptious Cod in Delish Sauce
53	Delish Baked dill Salmon
54	Prawn garlic Fried "Rice"
55	Lemon and Thyme Super Salmon
56	Delicious Salmon in Herb Crust
57	Salmon Mustard Delish
58	Sexy Spicy Salmon
59	Mouthwatering Stuffed Salmon
60	Spectacular Salmon
61	Creamy Coconut Salmon
62	Salmon Dill Bonanza
63	Sexy Shrimp Cocktail
64	Gambas al Ajillo--Sizzling Garlic Shrimp
65	Garlic Lemon Shrimp bonanza

66	Courgette pesto and Shrimp
67	Easy Shrimp Stir Fry
68	Delectable Shrimp Scampi
69	Citrus Shrimp Delux
70	Sexy Garlic Shrimp
71	Shrimp Cakes Delux
72	Shrimp Spinach Spectacular
73	Prawn Salad Boats
74	Cheeky Curry Shrimp
75	Courgette Shrimp Coquettes
76	Sexy Shrimp on Sticks
77	Delicious Fish Stir Fry
78	Sexy Shrimp with Delish Veggie Stir Fry

SALAD – ANIMAL PROTEIN

79	Skinny Delicious Slaw
80	Turkey Eastern Surprise
81	Mediterranean Turkey Delish Salad
82	Skinny Delicious Turkey Divine
83	Chicken Basil Avo Salad
84	Skinny Chicken salad
85	Turkey Taco Salad
86	Cheeky Turkey Salad
87	Macadamia Chicken Salad
88	Rosy Chicken Supreme salad
89	Turkey Sprouts Salad
90	Delicious Chicken Salad

91	Avocado Tuna Salad
92	Classic Tuna Salad
93	Artichoke Tuna Delight
94	Tasty Tuna Stuffed Tomato
95	Advanced Avocado Tuna Salad
96	Sexy Italian Tuna Salad
97	Divine Chicken or Turkey and Baby Bok Choy Salad
98	Mediterranean Medley Salad
99	Spicy Eastern salad
100	Basil Avocado Bonanza Salad
101	Chinese Divine Salad
102	Divinely Delish Salad Surprise
103	Avocado Salad with Cilantro and Lime
104	Mexican Medley Salad
105	Macadamia Nut Chicken/Turkey Salad
106	Red Cabbage Bonanza Salad
107	Spectacular Sprouts Salad
108	Avocado Egg Salad
109	Avocado Divine Salad
110	Classic Waldorf Salad
111	Artichoke Heart & Turkey Salad Radicchio Cups
112	Tempting Tuna Stuffed Tomato
113	Incredibly Delish Avocado Tuna Salad
114	Italian Tuna Bonanza Salad
115	Asian Aspiration Salad

116   Tasty Carrot Salad

117   Creamy Carrot Salad

PURE VEGETABLES – PLEASE ADD ANY RAW NUTS and/or AVOCADO TO OBTAIN THE KETO FAT REQUIREMENT ON ALL THESE RECIPES!

118   Vegetarian Curry with Squash

119   Saucy Gratin with Creamy Cauliflower Bonanza

120   Egg Bok Choy and Basil Stir-Fry

121   Skinny Eggie Vegetable Stir Fry

122   Rucola Salad

123   Tasty Spring Salad

124   Spinach and Dandelion Pomegranate Salad

125   Pure Delish Spinach Salad

126   Sexy Salsa Salad

127   Eastern Avo Salad

128   Curry Coconut Salad

129   Jalapeno Salsa

130   Beet Sprout Divine Salad

131   Divine Carrot Salad

132   Cauliflower Couscous

133   Mouthwatering Mushroom Salad

134   Skinny Sweet Potato Salad

DESERTS

135   Fabulous Brownie Treats

136	Rose Banana Delicious Brownies
137	Pristine Pumpkin Divine
138	Secret Brownies
139	Spectacular Spinach Brownies
140	Choco-coco brownies
141	Coco – walnut Brownie Bites
142	Best Ever Banana Surprise Cake
143	Choco Cookie Delight
144	Choco triple delight
145	Peach and Almond Cake
146	Apple Cinnamon Walnut Bonanza
147	Chestnut- Cacao Cake
148	Extra Dark Choco Delight
149	Nut Butter Truffles
150	Fetching Fudge
151	Choco – Almond Delights
152	Chococups
153	Choco Coco Cookies
154	Apple Spice Spectacular
155	Absolute Almond bites
156	Eastern Spice Delights
157	Berry Ice Cream and Almond delight
158	Creamy Caramely IceCream
159	Cheeky Cherry Ice
160	Choco - Coconut Berry Ice

161 Creamy Berrie Pie

162 Peachy Creamy Peaches

163 Spiced Apple Bake

164 Sexy Dessert Pan

165 Pretty Pumpkin Delights

166 Macadamia Pineapple Bonanza

167 Lemonny Lemon Delights

SMOOTHIES

168 Gorgeous Berry Smoothie

169 Tempting Coconut Berry Smoothie

170 Volumptious Vanilla Hot Drink

171 Almond Butter Smoothies

172 Choco Walnut Delight

173 Raspberry Hemp Smoothie

174 Choco Banana Smoothie

175 Blueberry Almond Smoothie

176 Hazelnut Butter and Banana Smoothie

177 Vanilla Blueberry Smoothie

178 Chocolate Raspberry Smoothie

179 Peach Smoothie

180 Zesty Citrus Smoothie

181 Apple Smoothie

182 Pineapple Smoothie

183 Strawberry Smoothie

184 Pineapple Coconut Delux Smoothie

185 Divine Vanilla Smoothie

186 CoCo Orange Delish Smoothie

187 Baby Kale Pineapple Smoothie

188 Sumptious Strawberry Coconut Smoothie

189 Blueberry Bonanza Smoothies

190 Divine Peach Coconut Smoothie

191 Tantalizing Key Lime Pie Smoothie

192 High Protein and Nutritional Delish Smoothie

193 Pineapple Protein Smoothie

194 Raspberry Coconut Smoothie

195 Ginger Carrot Protein Smoothie

SNACKS

196 Delish Banana Nut Muffins

197 Delightful Cinnamon Apple Muffins

198 Healthy Breakfast Bonanza Muffins

199 Perfect Pumpkin Seeds

200 Gorgeous Spicy Nuts

201 Krunchy Yummy Kale Chips

202 Delicious Cinnamon Apple Chips

203 Gummy Citrus Snack

204 Skinny Veggie Dip

205 Divine Butternut Chips

206 Outstanding Orange Skinny Snack

207 Spicy Pumpkin Seed Bonanza

208 Delectable Chocolate-Frosted Doughnuts

209	Eggplant Divine
210	Choco Apple Nachos
211	Skinny Delicious Snack Bars
212	Pumpkin Vanilla Delight
213	Skinny Quicky Crackers
214	Delectable Parsnip Chips
215	Spicy Crunchy Skinny Snack
216	Raw Hemp Kale Bars
217	Skinny Trail Mix
218	Anti-Aging Fruit Delights
219	Paleo Rosemary Sweet Potato Crunches
220	Apple Peach skinny Bars
221	Spicy Fried Almonds
222	Zucchini Avocado Hummus
223	Skinny Power Snack
224	Skinny Salsa - *Add any of the crunchy chip recipes mentioned in this book*
225	Divine Turkey Stuffed Tomatoes
226	Curried Nutty Delish
227	Skinny Chips
228	Zesty Zucchini Pesto Roll-ups
229	Butternut Squash-raw Veggie Dip
230	Skinny Power Balls
231	Chocolate Goji Skinny Bars
232	Delish Cashew Butter Treats

SOUPS

233   Roasted Tasty Tomato Soup

234   Thai Coconut Turkey Soup

235   Cheeky Chicken Soup

236   Triple Squash Delight Soup

237   Ginger Carrot Delight Soup

238   Wonderful Watercress Soup

239   Curried Butternut Soup

240   Celery Cashew Cream Soup

241   Mighty Andalusian Gazpacho

242   Munchy Mushroom Soup

243   Tempting Tomato Basil Soup

244   Healing Chicken/Turkey Vegetable Soup

245   Sumptuous Saffron Turkey Cauliflower Soup

246   Delicious Masala Soup

247   Creamy Chicken Soup

248   Delicious Lemon-Garlic Soup

249   Turkey Squash Soup

250   Roasted Winter Vegetable Turkey Soup

251   Zucchini Fish Soup Delight!

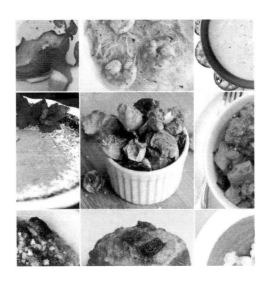

Chapter 10

The PKE DIET REVOLUTION Plan

How the Epigenetic Weight Loss Plan Works: The Basics

The Plan is a 3 week life changing eating program, meaning that you will be eating pure, healthy Paleo Epigenetic options for a full 3 week period to achieve the maximum permanent benefits. You will not be hungry!

If you would like to learn more about the New Paleo PKE Diet, we suggest you download the initial book in this series

PALEO EPIGENETIC RECIPES

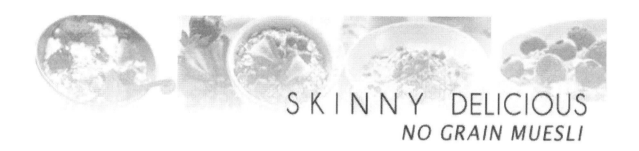

Paleo Epigenetic Breakfasts (Grain Free)

1. Gutsy Granola

Ingredients:
1 cup cashews
3/4 cup almonds
1/4 cup pumpkin seeds, shelled
1/4 cup sunflower seeds, shelled
1/2 cup unsweetened coconut flakes
1/4 cup coconut oil
Stevia to taste
1 tsp vanilla
low sodium salt to taste

Instructions:
Preheat oven to 300 degrees F. Line a baking sheet with parchment paper. Place the cashews, almonds, coconut flakes and pumpkin seeds into a blender and pulse to break the mixture into smaller pieces.

In a large microwave-safe bowl, melt the coconut oil, vanilla, and stevia together for 40-50 seconds. Add in the mixture from the blender and the sunflower seeds, and stir to coat.

Spread the mixture out onto the baking sheet and cook for 20-25 minutes, stirring once, until the mixture is lightly browned. Remove from heat. Add low sodium salt.

Press the granola mixture together to form a flat, even surface. Cool for about 15 minutes, and then break into pieces.

2. Spicy Granola

Ingredients:
1 ½ cups almond flour
1/3 cup coconut oil
2 tsp cinnamon
2 tsp nutmeg
2 tsp vanilla extract
½ cup walnuts
½ cup coconut flakes
¼ cup hemp seeds
low sodium salt, to taste

Instructions:
Preheat oven to 275 degrees Fahrenheit.

Combine all ingredients in a large mixing bowl and mix well… melt down the coconut oil a little bit before adding it

Spread mixture into one flat layer on a greased baking sheet.

Bake for 40-50 minutes, or until mixture is toasted to your liking.

Remove from oven and allow to cool before serving, then transfer into a plastic container.

3. High Protein Breakfast Gold

Ingredients:
1/2 cup (c). Flax-Meal, golden
1/2 c. Chia seed
Stevia liquid to taste
2 tbs. dark ground cinnamon
1 tbs. hemp protein powder
2 tbs. coconut oil, melted
1 tsp. vanilla extract
3/4 c. + 2 tbs. hot water

Instructions:

Begin to spread the dough out until its super thin, onto a parchment paper lined cookie sheet. Bake at 325 for 15 minutes, then drop it down to 300 and leave for 30 minutes.

Before dropping it, pull out the sheet and cut it. Put it back into the oven exactly like this, don't separate the pieces.

When the 30 minutes are up, pull it out and separate the pieces. Drop the pieces to 200 degrees F for 1 hour. They will be completely dried out at this point. Enjoy with almond or other nut milk!

4. Apple Breakfast Dream

Ingredients:
2 Cup (C) raw walnuts
1 C raw macadamia nuts
2 apples, peeled and diced
1 Tbsp coconut oil
1 Tbsp ground cinnamon
2 C almond milk
1 14 oz can full fat coconut milk

Instructions:
Combine nuts and dates in a food processor until ground into a fine meal, about 1 minute; set aside.

Saute apples over medium heat in coconut oil until lightly browned, about 5 minutes.

Add nut mixture and cinnamon to apples and stir to incorporate, about 1 minute.

Reduce heat to low and add coconut and almond milk.

Stirring occasionally, let mixture cook uncovered until thickened, about 25 minutes.

5. Divine Protein Muesli

Ingredients:
1 cup unsweetened unsulfured coconut flakes
1 tbsp chopped walnuts
1 tbsp raw almonds (~10)
1 tbsp chocolate chips (dark and sugar free)
1/2 tsp cinnamon
1 cup unsweetened almond milk
1 scoop hemp protein

Instructions:
In a medium bowl layer coconut flakes, walnuts, almonds and chocolate chips.

Sprinkle with cinnamon.

Pour cold almond milk over the muesli and eat with a spoon.

6. Ultimate Skinny Granola

Ingredients:
1 cup of unsweetened coconut milk or unsweetened almond milk
Stevia liquid to taste
1 tablespooneach of unsalted …
pecan pieces
walnut pieces
almonds
pistachios
raw pine nuts
raw sunflower/safflower seeds
raw pumpkin seeds
2 Tablespoons of frozen or fresh berry selection (e.g. blueberries, blackberries, raspberries, strawberries, or other kinds etc)

Instructions:
Put all the nuts & seeds in a breakfast bowl.

add a few drops of pure liquid stevia and stir it well in.

Add the berries and milk.

If using frozen berries, wait for 2-3 minutes for them to get warmer.

The berries will now release some color into the milk, making it look really interesting. Enjoy!

7. Apple Chia Delight

Ingredients:
2c organic chia seeds (black or white)
1c organic hemp hearts
1/2 chopped fresh apple
2tbsp real cinnamon
1 tsp low sodium salt
optional: 1/2c chopped nuts of your choice

Instructions:
Throw all of this together, mix it up, and enjoy with almond milk. Stevia to taste.

8. Tasty Apple Almond Coconut Medley

Ingredients:
one-half apple cored and roughly diced
handful of sliced almonds
handful of unsweetened coconut
generous dose of cinnamon
1 pinch of low sodium salt

Instructions:
Pulse in the food processor to desired consistency–smaller is better for the little ones! Serve with almond milk, or creamy coconut milk.

9. Choco Nut Skinny Muesli Balls

Ingredients:
1 cup of raw almonds
1 Tablespoon of coconut oil
¼ teaspoon low sodium salt
2 Tablespoon Coconut flour
1 egg white
2 Tablespoon plus 1 teaspoon of Cacao powder
pure liquid stevia to taste

Instructions:

First grind the almonds in a food processor or blender until you have a flour.

Add the ground almonds, low sodium salt, coconut flour, egg white, pure liquid stevia and cacao power to a bowl and mix with a spoon until you have a dough.

Either:

a) Place the dough onto a piece of parchment paper. Place a second piece of parchment paper over the top and roll it until it is ¼" thick. With a wet knife, score it into 1" squares. Place the parchment paper on a baking sheet when finished.

Or

b) Take a small pinch of the dough and roll into a ¼ round ball and set on a baking sheet lined with parchment paper.

Turn on your oven and set to 350 degrees and bake for 15 - 18 minutes for cereal balls or bake for 8 to 12 minutes for flat cereal.

Remove from the oven and let cool on the pan.

Top with your favorite nut or seed milk and enjoy!

10. Sweetie Skinny Crackers

Ingredients:
1 egg
pure liquid stevia to taste
1 Tbspn coconut oil, melted
1.5 cups almond flour
.5 cup coconut flour
1 teaspoon cinnamon

Instructions:
Preheat oven to 350°

In a large bowl, whisk together the egg, pure liquid stevia and melted coconut oil

Add the coconut and almond flour and stir to combine.

Give the dough a couple of kneads so it's well incorporated.

Turn the dough onto a piece of parchment paper and flatten a bit with your hands.

Place another piece of parchment on top and roll out with a rolling pin until it's about 1/8 inch thick.

Remove the top piece of parchment and cut the dough into 1/4 inch squares for cereal, and about 2"x3" for crackers

Sprinkle the cinnamon into the dough mixture.

Slide the dough with the bottom parchment paper onto a baking sheet and bake for 15 minutes.

Turn down the oven to 325° and bake for another 10-15 minutes, or until the cereal / crackers are crisp.

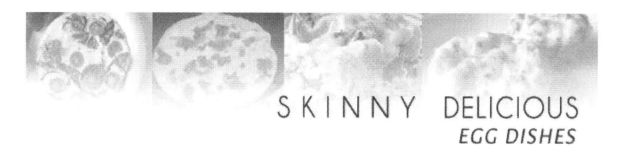

SKINNY DELICIOUS
EGG DISHES

Paleo Epigenetic Egg Meals

1. Scrambled Eggs with Chilli

Ingredients:
4 fresh green chillies with skins removed
2 tablespoons (30g or 1 oz) coconut oil
    1 small onion, peeled and finely chopped
6 eggs
1/4 cup (62ml or 2 fl oz) coconut milk
low sodium salt to taste

Instructions:
After removing chilli skins, remove and discard seeds and finely chop remaining chilli.

Beat eggs, coconut milk and salt in a bowl and set aside.

Heat oil in a medium size saucepan over a medium heat.

Reduce heat to low and add egg mixture to saucepan and mix well.

Scatter chilies over mixture.

Cook over a low heat until eggs are cooked.

Serves 4. Serve hot.

2. Basil and Walnut Eggs Divine

Ingredients:
3 organic eggs
1/2 cup fresh basil, chopped
1/3 cup walnuts, chopped
salt and pepper

Instructions:

Whisk eggs in a bowl then place in a frying pan on medium heat, stirring constantly.

When the eggs are almost cooked, add the basil and continue cooking for a further 1 minute or until eggs are fully cooked.

Add salt and pepper to taste.

Remove from heat and stir in the walnuts before serving.

3. Spicy Scrambled Eggs

Ingredients:
1 tablespoon extra virgin olive oil
1 red onion, finely chopped
1 medium green pepper, cored, seeded, and finely chopped
1 chilli, seeded and cut into thin strips
3 ripe tomatoes, peeled, seeded, and chopped
Salt and freshly ground black pepper
4 large organic eggs

Instructions:

Heat the olive oil in a large, heavy, preferably nonstick skillet over medium heat.

Add the onion and cook until soft, 6 to 7 minutes.

Add the pepper and chilli and continue cooking until soft, another 4 to 5 minutes.

Add in the tomatoes, and salt and pepper to taste and cook uncovered, over low heat for 10 minutes.

Add the eggs, stirring them into the mixture to distribute.

Cover the skillet and cook until the eggs are set but still fluffy and tender, about 7 to 8 minutes. Divide between 4 plates and serve.

4. Spicy India Omelet

Ingredients:
3 Eggs
1 Onion, chopped
4 Green Chilli (optional)
1/4 cup Coconut grated
Low sodium Salt asrequired
1 tblspoon olive oil

Instructions:
Beat the Eggs severely.

Mix chopped onion, rounded green chilli, salt and grated coconuts with eggs.

Heat oil on a medium-low heat, in a pan.

Pour the mixture in the form of pancakes and cook it on the both sides.

5. Spectacular Spinach Omelet

Ingredients:
2 eggs
1.5 cups raw spinach
coconut oil, about 1 tbsp
1/3 c tomatoes and onion salsa (lightly fried in pan)
1 tbsp fresh cilantro

Instructions:

Melt coconut oil on medium in frying pan. Add spinach, cook until mostly wilted. Beat eggs and add to pan.

Flip once the egg sets around the edge. When it's almost done add the salsa on top just to warm it. Move to plate and add cilantro. Serves one.

6. Blushing Blueberry Omelet

Ingredients:
2 eggs
1 tsp. vanilla extract
coconut oil
1/2 c. blueberries
Stevia to taste

Instructions:

Lightly beat two eggs and vanilla extract in a bowl. Heat 6" non-stick pan over medium heat.

While pan is heating, heat half the blueberries in a saucepan until juices flow.

Add coconut oil to non-stick pan and coat evenly.

When thoroughly heated, add egg mixture. Turn once and let sit.

When eggs are about 70% settled, turn again. There should be a nice crispy layer around the side of the pan.

When it starts to separate from the side, add fresh and cooked blueberries to omelet, reserving a few for garnish.

Crispy layer should really be pulling away from pan now.

Use a fork to help fold the omelet over. Slide on to plate, top with reserved blueberry filling, and enjoy!

7. Mediterranean Supercharger Omelet with Fennel and Dill

Ingredients:
2 tablespoons olive oil, divided
2 cups thinly sliced fresh fennel bulb, fronds chopped and reserved
8 cherry tomatoes
5 large eggs, beaten to blend with 1/4 teaspoon salt and 1/4 teaspoon ground black pepper
1 1/2 tablespoons chopped fresh dill

Instructions:

Add remaining 1 tablespoon oil to same skillet; heat over medium-high heat.

Add beaten eggs and cook until eggs are just set in center, tilting skillet and lifting edges of omelet with spatula to let uncooked portion flow underneath, about 3 minutes.

Top with fennel mixture. Sprinkle dill over.

Using spatula, fold uncovered half of omelet over; slide onto plate.

Garnish with chopped fennel and serve.

8. Outstanding Veggie Omelette

Ingredients:
3 eggs, beaten
1 carrot, matchstick cut
3 scallions, diagonal sliced
1 handful tiny broccoli florets or whatever leftover veggies you have
Bits of leftover cooked turkey
Safflower oil
Low sodium salt

Instructions:
Heat oil in a wok or large cast iron skillet over medium heat, until hot enough to sizzle a drop of water.

Add broccoli and carrots, stir fry 2 min. until soft.

Add cooked turkey, stir fry 1 min. until heated through. Add scallions and eggs, scramble. Add salt to taste. Serve.

9. Spicy Spinach Bake

Ingredients:
6 eggs
1 bunch fresh spinach chopped (a box of frozen will do if you do not have fresh)
1/2 tsp hot pepper flakes
Olive oil
Low sodium Salt and pepper

Instructions:
Scramble the eggs in a bowl. Add the spinach, low sodium salt and pepper.

Scramble together. Heat a large non-stick skillet with about 1/2 cup olive oil.

When the oil is hot put the hot pepper flakes in then pour the mixture in. When it starts to cook on the bottom, flip it over

Take it out when it is medium scrambled. Let cool and eat.

10. Delish Veggie Hash With Eggs

Ingredients:
2 tablespoon extra virgin olive oil
2 garlic cloves, minced
1/4 cup sweet white onion, chopped
1 cup yellow squash, chopped
1/2 cup mushroom, sliced
Low sodium salt and pepper
1 cup cherry tomatoes, halved
1 cup fresh spinach, chopped
4 eggs, poached or cooked any style
You can substitute the squash with whatever vegetables you have

Instructions:
Heat large non-stick skillet over medium heat. Add olive oil to pan.

Add garlic and onion and saute for 2 minutes, then add chopped squash or your favorite vegetable, cook for 2 more minutes, then add mushrooms. Cook for 5-minutes or until almost compete.

At this point add low sodium salt and pepper, then add tomatoes and spinach and cook until spinach wilts. Drain well before plating.

While finishing this prepare eggs to your liking in another pan.

To serve, drained hash mixture to and then add to individual plates. On top of hash add 2 cooked eggs per person.

11. Spectacular Eggie Salsa

Ingredients:
2 pounds fresh ripe tomatoes, peeled and coarsely chopped
2 to 3 serrano or jalapeño chiles, seeded for a milder sauce, and chopped
2 garlic cloves, peeled, halved, green shoots removed
1/2 small onion, chopped
2 tablespoons oil
Low sodium salt to taste
4 to 8 eggs (to taste)
Chopped cilantro for garnish

Instructions:

Place the tomatoes, chilies, garlic and onion in a blender and puree, retaining a bit of texture.

Heat 1 tablespoon of the oil over high heat in a large, heavy nonstick skillet, until a drop of puree will sizzle when it hits the pan.

Add the puree and cook, stirring, for four to ten minutes, until the sauce thickens, darkens and leaves a trough when you run a spoon down the middle of the pan. It should just begin to stick to the pan.

Season to taste with salt, and remove from the heat. Keep warm while you fry the eggs.

Warm four plates. Fry the eggs in a heavy skillet over medium-high heat.

 Use the remaining tablespoon of oil if necessary. Cook them sunny side up, until the whites are solid but the yolks still runny.

Season with salt and pepper, and turn off the heat. Place one or two fried eggs on each plate.

Spoon the hot salsa over the whites of the eggs, leaving the yolks exposed if possible. Sprinkle with cilantro and serve.

12. Mushrooms, Eggs and Onion Bonanza

Ingredients:
1 medium onion, finely diced
1/4 cup coconut oil
10-12 medium white mushrooms, finely chopped
12 hard boiled eggs, peeled and finely chopped
Freshly ground black pepper to taste

Instructions:
Saute the onion in coconut oil until golden brown.

Add the mushrooms and saute another 5 minutes or so, stirring frequently, until mushrooms are softened and turned dark.

Remove from heat and let cool.

Mix together with the eggs and pepper. Chill until ready to serve.

13. Avocado and Shrimp Omelet

Ingredients:
6 eggs
2 Tbsp. chopped parsley
2 Tbsp. lemon juice, divided
1/4 tsp. salt
1/8 tsp. cayenne pepper
1 large* ripe avocado, diced
1 1/2 Tbsp. avocado oil
3 oz. bay shrimp
3 parsley sprigs

Instructions:

Beat together eggs, parsley, 3/4 of the lemon juice, salt, and cayenne pepper; reserve.

Gently toss avocado with remaining lemon juice; reserve.

Heat oil in an omelet pan. (Use a large omelet pan for four or more servings.)

Pour egg mixture into pan.

Cook over medium heat, lifting edges and tilting pan to allow uncooked egg to run under, until set but still moist on top.

Scatter reserved avocado and shrimp over omelet.

Fold omelet in half; heat another minute or two.

Slide onto a warmed serving plate; garnish with parsley sprigs.

To serve, cut omelet into wedges.

14. Delish Veggie Breakfast Peppers

Ingredients:
2 bell peppers – your choice of color
4 eggs
1 cup white mushrooms
1 cup broccoli
¼ tsp cayenne pepper
low sodium salt and pepper, to taste

Instructions:
Preheat oven to 375 degrees Fahrenheit.

Dice up your vegetables of choice.

In a medium sized bowl, mix eggs, low sodium salt, pepper, cayenne pepper, and vegetables.

Cut peppers into equal halves. A tip:

Core the peppers so that they're clean enough to add the filling.

Pour a quarter of the egg / vegetable mix into each pepper halve, adding more vegetables to the top to fill in any empty space.

Place on baking sheet and cook approximately 35 minutes.

15. Breakfast Mexicana

Ingredients:
For the tortillas:
2 eggs
2 egg whites
1/2 cup water
4 tsp ground flaxseed
Pinch of low sodium salt

For the filling:
1 avocado, diced
1/4 cup red bell pepper, finely diced
1/4 cup onion, finely diced
1/4 cup baked cod or other protein
Handful of spinach leaves
1 tsp coconut oil

Instructions:

In a small bowl, whisk together the ingredients for the tortilla. Preheat the oven

Heat a 10-inch non-stick skillet over medium heat and coat well with coconut oil spray.

Pour half of the tortilla mixture into the pan and swirl to evenly distribute.

Using a metal spatula, loosen the edges of the tortilla from the pan.

Cook a couple of minutes until golden brown on the bottom, and then carefully slide the spatula under the tortilla to loosen it from the bottom of the pan. Do not flip yet.

Place the pan under the broiler for 3-4 minutes until the tortilla gets a little bubbly.

Remove the tortilla from the pan, setting on a piece of aluminum foil. Repeat with other half of tortilla mixture.

After the tortillas are done broiling, preheat the oven to 400 degrees F. In a separate small pan, heat the coconut oil over medium heat.

Add the onions and peppers and sauté for 5-8 minutes, until soft. Add the spinach into the pan and wilt.

Place all of the fillings down the center of the tortillas and wrap tightly. Place into the oven for 5-8 minutes to set. It's so delish!

16. Zucchini Casserole

Ingredients:
3 large zucchini
1/2 red onion, chopped
1/2 cup mushrooms
5 eggs
1 tsp low sodium salt
Freshly ground black pepper, to taste

Instructions:
Preheat oven to 375 degrees F..

Grate all of the zucchini and put into a large bowl.

In a separate bowl, beat the eggs with low sodium salt and pepper.

Combine all of the ingredients, in the large bowl and mix together. You want to have enough eggs to coat the whole mixture.

Warm about a 1/2 tablespoon of olive oil in the skillet over medium heat.

Add the zucchini mixture into the pan. Cover and cook about 5 minutes until the eggs start to set on the bottom.

Transfer to the oven and bake for 12-15 minutes, until the eggs are firm. Remove and let rest for 5-10 minutes, then serve.

17. Blueberry Nut Casserole

Ingredients:
Crush one cup almonds, walnuts and pecans with one teaspoon olive oil and bake
    in the oven at 200 for 20 minutes
2 cups frozen blueberries
5 eggs
1 cup almond milk
Stevia to taste
1 tsp vanilla extract
1 tsp cinnamon
Pinch of nutmeg

Instructions:

Preheat the oven to 350 degrees F. Grease an 8x8-inch baking dish with coconut oil spray. Place the nut crust and blueberries into the dish.

Whisk together the eggs, almond milk, stevia, vanilla, and cinnamon in a medium bowl.

Pour the egg mixture over the crust and blueberries. Lightly stir to coat.

Bake for 35-45 minutes. Remove from the oven and allow the casserole to rest for 15 minutes before serving.

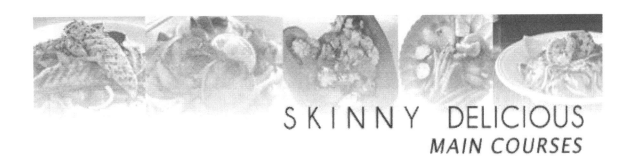

SKINNY DELICIOUS
MAIN COURSES

Paleo Epigenetic Main Meals (Lunch or Dinner)

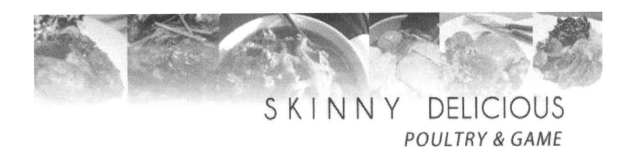

SKINNY DELICIOUS
POULTRY & GAME

Paleo Epigenetic Poultry & Game

1. Spicy Turkey Stir Fry

Ingredients:
2 lbs. boneless skinless chicken or turkey breasts, cut into 1-inch slices
2 tbsp coconut oil
1 tsp cumin seeds
1/2 each green, red, and orange bell pepper, thinly sliced
1 tsp garam masala
2 tsp freshly ground pepper
low sodium salt, to taste
Scallions, for garnish

For the marinade:
1/2 cup coconut cream
1 clove garlic, minced
1 tsp ginger, minced
1 tbsp freshly ground pepper
2 tsp low sodium salt
1/4 tsp turmeric

Instructions:

Place all of the marinade ingredients into a Ziploc bag. Add the chicken, close the bag, and shake to coat.

Marinate in the refrigerator for at least 30 minutes, or up to 6 hours.

In a wok or large sauté pan, melt the coconut oil over medium-high heat. Add the cumin seeds and cook for 2-3 minutes.

Add the marinated chicken and let cook for 5 minutes. Stir the chicken until it begins to brown, and then add the peppers, garam masala, and freshly ground pepper.

Sprinkle with low sodium salt. Cook for 4-5 minutes, stirring regularly, or until the bell pepper is cooked to desired doneness. Serve hot.

2. Turkey and Kale Pasta Casserole

Ingredients:
1 lb. Turkey breast
1 medium spaghetti squash, halved and seeded
Extra virgin olive oil, for drizzling
1 large bunch of kale, de-stemmed, and chopped
1/2 red onion, sliced thin
1/3 cup chicken broth
1/2 cup coconut milk
1 clove garlic, minced
2 tsp Italian seasoning – salt free
low sodium salt and freshly ground pepper, to taste

Instructions:

Preheat the oven to 400 degrees F. Place the squash in the microwave for 3-4 minutes to soften.

Using a sharp knife, cut the squash in half lengthwise. Scoop out the seeds and discard. Place the halves, with the cut side up, on a rimmed baking sheet.

Drizzle with olive oil and sprinkle with low sodium salt and pepper. Roast in the oven for 45-50 minutes, until you can poke the squash easily with a fork.

Let it cool until you can handle it safely. Then scrape the insides with a fork to shred the squash into strands.

Meanwhile, melt the coconut oil in a large oven-safe skillet over medium heat.

Add the turkey breast and brown. Once cooked through, remove to a plate. In the same skillet, add the onion and sauté for 3-4 minutes.

Next add the garlic, Italian seasoning, and kale and cook for 2-3 minutes to slightly wilt the kale.

Pour in the chicken broth and coconut milk and simmer for an additional 2-3 minutes. Remove from heat.

Stir in the cooked turkey. Add the spaghetti squash into the skillet and stir well to combine.

Bake for 15-18 minutes, until the top has slightly browned. Serve hot.

3. Roasted Lemon Herb Chicken

Ingredients:
12 total pieces bone-in chicken thighs and legs
1 medium onion, thinly sliced
1 tbsp dried rosemary
1 tsp dried thyme
1 lemon, sliced thin
1 orange, sliced thin

For the marinade:
5 tbsp extra virgin olive oil
6 cloves garlic, minced
Stevia to taste
Juice of 1 lemon
Juice of 1 orange
1 tbsp Italian seasoning – salt free
1 tsp onion powder
Dash of red pepper flakes
low sodium salt and freshly ground pepper, to taste

Instructions:

Whisk together all of the marinade ingredients in a small bowl. Place the chicken in a baking dish (or a large Ziploc bag) and pour the marinade over it. Marinate for 3 hours to overnight.

Preheat the oven to 400 degrees F. Place the chicken in a baking dish and arrange with the onion, orange, and lemon slices.

Sprinkle with thyme, rosemary, low sodium salt and pepper. Cover with aluminum foil and bake for 30 minutes.

Remove the foil, baste the chicken, and bake for another 30 minutes uncovered, until the chicken is cooked through.

4. Basil Turkey with Roasted Tomatoes

Ingredients:
2 turkey breasts
1 cup mushrooms, chopped
1/2 medium onion, chopped
1-2 tbsp extra virgin olive oil
Half cup thinly sliced fresh basil
low sodium salt and pepper, to taste
1 pint cherry tomatoes
Stevia to taste
Fresh parsley, for garnish

Instructions:
Preheat the oven to 400 degrees F. Place the tomatoes on a baking sheet and drizzle with olive oil and stevia. Sprinkle with low sodium salt and pepper and toss to coat evenly. Bake for 15-20 minutes until soft.

While the tomatoes are roasting, heat one tablespoon of olive oil in a large pan over low heat. Add the onions and mushrooms and cook for 10-12 minutes to soften and caramelize, stirring regularly. Clear a space for the chicken.

Season the turkey with low sodium salt and pepper and then place it in the pan. Simmer for 15 minutes or until the chicken is cooked through. Every 5 minutes or so, spoon the sauce in the pan over the turkey.

To assemble, divide the tomatoes between two plates. Place one turkey breast on each and then spoon the onions, mushrooms, and pan drippings over the turkey. Garnish with parsley.

5. Roasted and Filled Tasty Bell Peppers

Ingredients:
5 large bell peppers
1 tbsp coconut oil
1/2 large onion, diced
1 tsp dried oregano
1/2 tsp low sodium salt
1 lb. ground turkey
1 large zucchini, halved and diced
3 tbsp tomato paste
Freshly ground black pepper, to taste
Fresh parsley, for serving

Instructions:
Preheat the oven to 350 degrees F. Coat a small baking dish with coconut oil spray. Bring a large pot of water to a boil. Cut the stems and very top of the peppers off, removing the seeds. Place in boiling water for 4-5 minutes. Remove from the water and drain face-down on a paper towel.

Heat the coconut oil in a large nonstick pan over medium heat. Add in the onion. Sauté for 3-4 minutes until the onion begins to soften. Stir in the ground turkey, oregano, low sodium salt, and pepper and cook until turkey is browned.

Add the zucchini to the skillet as the turkey finishes cooking. Cook everything together until the zucchini is soft, and then drain any juices from the pan.

Remove the pan from heat and stir in the tomato paste. Bake for 15 minutes.

6. Chili-Garlic Ostrich or Venison Skewers

Ingredients:
6 Wooden Skewers, soaked in cold water for 30 minutes
2 Ostrich or Venison, diced
1 tbsp. Olive Oil
1 tsp. Red Chilies, seeds removed & finely chopped
4 Garlic Cloves, minced
6 tbsp. fresh lemon juice

Instructions:
Preheat oven to 350 F or preheat barbeque grill on high heat.

To make sauce, combine the oil, chilies, garlic, and lemon juice in a small bowl. Set aside for a few minutes.

Thread diced meat onto skewers and place on an oven tray lined with baking paper.

Pour chili and garlic sauce over the chicken, coating well.

Bake in the oven for 30-40 minutes or until chicken is cooked. If cooking on a grill, cook meat or poultry for 5-6 minutes on each side.

Eat with any of the delicious salad recipes.

7. Creamy Chicken Casserole

Ingredients:
2 cups cubed cooked chicken
1 1/2 cups cooked butternut squash
1/2 cup coconut cream,
1/4 cup coconut oil, melted
1 heaping cup green peas, fresh or frozen
1 tbsp apple cider vinegar
1/2 tsp low sodium salt
1/2 tsp oregano
1/2 tsp thyme
1 tbsp fresh parsley

Instructions:

In a large bowl, mash the butternut squash. Stir in the coconut cream, oil, vinegar, low sodium salt, oregano, and thyme.

Once everything is combined, add in chicken and peas.

Place the mixture into a large saucepan and cook over medium heat for 5-8 minutes.

Top with fresh parsley and serve warm.

8. Spectacular Spaghetti and Delish Turkey Balls

Ingredients:
1 spaghetti squash
Extra virgin olive oil,
low sodium salt and pepper
1 tsp dried or fresh oregano

For the sauce:
1 lb ground turkey
1 small onion, chopped
4 cloves garlic, minced
1 tbsp coconut oil
1 tomato, chopped
1/2 jar of tomato sauce
1 tbsp Italian seasoning
low sodium salt and pepper to taste
Fresh basil

Instructions:

Preheat oven to 400 degrees F. Using a sharp knife, cut the squash in half lengthwise. Scoop out the seeds and discard.

Place the halves with the cut side up on a rimmed baking sheet. Drizzle with olive oil and season with low sodium salt, pepper, and oregano. Roast the squash in the oven for 40-45 minutes, until you can poke the squash easily with a fork.

Let it cool until you can handle it safely. Then scrape the insides with a fork to shred the squash into strands.

While the spaghetti squash is roasting, melt coconut oil in a large skillet over medium heat.

Add chopped onion and garlic and cook for 4-5 minutes. Add ground turkey and brown the meat, stirring occasionally. Season with low sodium salt and pepper.

Add the chopped tomato, tomato sauce, and Italian seasoning and stir to combine. Simmer on low heat, stirring occasionally, while the spaghetti squash finishes roasting. Serve over spaghetti squash with basil for garnish.

9. Sensational Courgette Pasta and Turkey Bolognaise

Ingredients:
4 medium zucchini

For the sauce:
1 lb ground turkey
1 small onion, chopped
4 cloves garlic, minced
1 tbsp coconut oil
1 tomato, chopped
1/2 jar of tomato sauce
1 tbsp Italian seasoning
low sodium salt and pepper to taste
Fresh basil, for garnish

Instructions:

Use a julienne peeler to slice the zucchini into noodles, stopping when you reach the seeds. Set aside.

If cooking zucchini noodles, simply add to a skillet and sauté over medium heat for 4-5 minutes.

Melt coconut oil in a large skillet over medium heat. Add chopped onion and garlic and cook for 4-5 minutes.

Add ground turkey and brown the meat, stirring occasionally. Season with low sodium salt and pepper.

Add the chopped tomato, tomato sauce, and Italian seasoning and stir to combine. Simmer on low heat, stirring occasionally.

Add the sauce to the noodles and ENJOY.

10. Tempting Turkey Spaghetti Squash Boats

Ingredients:
1 medium spaghetti squash or 2 small spaghetti squash
1 1/2 lbs. Turkey mashed
1 yellow onion, diced
4 cloves garlic, minced
1 bunch kale
3 tbsp extra virgin olive oil, plus more for drizzling
low sodium salt and pepper
2 tbsp pine nuts, roasted
2 tbsp fresh parsley, chopped

Instructions:
Preheat the oven to 400 degrees F. Place squash in the microwave for 3-4 minutes to soften. Using a sharp knife cut the squash in half lengthwise. Scoop out the seeds and discard.

Place the halves, with the cut side up, on a rimmed baking sheet. Drizzle with olive oil and sprinkle with low sodium salt and pepper.

Roast in the oven for 45-50 minutes, until you can poke the squash easily with a fork. Let cool until you can handle it safely.

Meanwhile, prepare the kale by removing the center stems and either tearing or cutting up the leaves. Heat the olive oil in a large skillet over medium heat.

Add the onion and garlic and sauté for 4-5 minutes. Add the turkey. Cook for 10-12 minutes, stirring regularly, until the turkey is browned and cooked through.

Add the kale and stir. Cook for a few minutes more to wilt the kale. Remove from heat and set aside.

Once cooled, scrape the insides of the spaghetti squash with a fork to shred the squash into strands. Transfer the strands into the skillet with the turkey and toss to combine.

Season to taste with low sodium salt and pepper. Divide the mixture among the squash shells, and then top with pine nuts and parsley to serve.

11. Delicious Turkey Veggie Lasagna

Ingredients:

For the meat sauce:
1 large yellow onion, coarsely chopped
2 cloves garlic, coarsely chopped
2 tbsp extra virgin olive oil
1 1/2 lbs. ground turkey
1/2 cup tomato paste
1/2 cup tomato sauce
1 cup red wine
1 bay leaf
3 sprigs thyme
low sodium salt and freshly ground pepper, to taste

For the lasagna:
1 eggplant, sliced lengthwise thinly
1 tsp low sodium salt
1 tbsp extra virgin olive oil
2 yellow squash, sliced thinly
1/2 cup torn fresh basil leaves
8 oz. white mushrooms, sliced
2 cups fresh spinach
2 large zucchini, sliced lengthwise into ribbons

For the topping:
1/2 head cauliflower
1 tbsp olive oil
1/2 tsp garlic powder
1/2 tsp low sodium salt
Freshly ground pepper, to taste

Instructions:

To make the meat sauce, place the onion and garlic in a food processor and pulse to finely chop.

Heat the olive oil in a heavy-bottomed saucepan over medium heat. Add the onion and garlic and season with low sodium salt and pepper. Cook for 12-15 minutes until beginning to brown, stirring frequently.

Add the turkey to the pot and season with low sodium salt and pepper.

Cook for 15 minutes until browned. Stir in the tomato paste and cook for 2-3 minutes. Add the red wine to the pan and cook for 5 more minutes.

Add the tomato sauce, bay leaf, and thyme to the pan. Bring to a simmer, and then add 1/2 cup water.

Cook at a low simmer for 1 hour, stirring occasionally and adding more water if necessary. Adjust seasonings to taste. Discard the bay leaf and thyme.

Preheat the oven to 350 degrees F. Sprinkle the eggplant with low sodium salt and set aside for 15 minutes to drain. Rinse and pat dry.

Heat one tablespoon of olive oil in a skillet over medium heat. Cook the eggplant for 2-3 minutes per side until golden.

Layer the lasagna in a baking dish. Start by layering the yellow squash as the base. Add one third of the meat sauce on top of that, then lay the eggplant slices, fresh basil, and mushrooms.

Next add the rest of the meat sauce, then the spinach, zucchini, and finally drizzle with olive oil and sprinkle with low sodium salt and pepper. Bake for 40-45 minutes.

While the lasagna is baking, place the cauliflower in a blender and process until it reaches a rice-like consistency.

Add to a skillet and sauté with the olive oil, garlic powder, low sodium salt, and pepper over medium heat.

Cook for 6-8 minutes until soft, adding a tablespoon of water if necessary. After the lasagna has cooked for 20 minutes, sprinkle with the cauliflower and return to the oven for the remaining cooking time. Serve hot.

12. Ostrich Steak or Venison with Divine Mustard Sauce and Roasted Tomatoes

Ingredients:
For the tomatoes:
2 pints cherry tomatoes, halved
2 tbsp extra virgin olive oil
Stevia to taste
low sodium salt and freshly ground pepper

For the cauliflower rice:
1/2 head of cauliflower, chopped coarsely
1/2 small onion, finely diced
1 tbsp coconut oil
1 tbsp fresh parsley, chopped
low sodium salt and freshly ground pepper, to taste

For the meat:
4 Ostrich or venison steaks
Extra virgin olive oil
low sodium salt and freshly ground pepper
Coconut oil, for the pan

For the sauce:
1/4 cup red onion, finely diced
1/4 cup apple cider vinegar
1 cup low sodium chicken stock
1 tbsp whole grain mustard
low sodium salt and freshly ground pepper, to taste

Instructions:

Preheat the oven to 400 degrees F. Place the tomatoes on a baking sheet and drizzle with olive oil and honey. Sprinkle with low sodium salt and pepper and toss to coat evenly. Bake for 15-20 minutes until soft.

While the tomatoes are roasting, prepare the cauliflower rice. Place the cauliflower into a food processor and pulse until reduced to the size of rice grains.

Melt the coconut oil in a nonstick skillet over medium heat. Add the onion and cook for 5-6 minutes until translucent. Stir in the cauliflower, season with low sodium salt and pepper, and cover. Cook for 7-10 minutes until the cauliflower has softened, and then toss with parsley.

To make the lamb, preheat the oven to 325 degrees F. Pat the ostrich or venison dry and rub with olive oil. Generously season both sides with low sodium salt and pepper.

Heat one tablespoon of coconut oil in a cast iron skillet. When the pan is hot, add to the pan and sear for 2-3 minutes on all sides until golden brown.

Place the skillet in the oven and bake for 5-8 minutes until the ostrich or venison reaches desired doneness. Let rest for 10 minutes before serving.

While the meat is resting, add the red onion to the skillet with the pan drippings from the lamb. Sauté for 3-4 minutes, then add the white wine vinegar.

Turn the heat to high and cook until the vinegar has mostly evaporated. Add the stock and bring to a boil, cooking until the sauce reduces by half.

Stir in the mustard, and season to taste with low sodium salt and pepper. Pour over ostrich or venison to serve.

13. Tantalizing Turkey Pepper Stir-fry

Ingredients:
2 bell peppers, sliced
1 cup broccoli florets
2 cooked and shredded turkey breasts
1/4 teaspoon chili powder
low sodium salt and pepper to taste
1 tablespoon coconut oil for frying

Instructions:
Add 1 tablespoon coconut oil into a frying pan on a medium heat.

Place the sliced bell peppers into the frying pan.

After the bell peppers soften, add in the cooked turkey meat.

Add in the chili powder, low sodium salt and pepper.

Mix well and stir-fry for a few more minutes.

14. Cheeky Chicken Stir Fry

Ingredients:
1 pound boneless, skinless chicken breast
2 tablespoons coconut oil
1 medium onion, finely chopped (about 1 cup)
2 heads broccoli, sliced into 3-inch spears (about 4 cups)
2 medium carrots, sliced (about 1 cup)
2 heads baby bok choy, sliced crosswise into 1-inch strips (about 1½ cups)
4 ounces shiitake mushrooms, stemmed and thinly sliced (about 1 cup)
1 small zucchini, sliced (about 1 cup)
½ teaspoon low sodium salt
Garlic powder to taste
1½ cups water

Instructions:

Rinse the chicken and pat dry. Cut into 1-inch cubes and transfer to a plate.

Heat the coconut oil in a large skillet over medium heat

Saute the onion for 8 to 10 minutes, until soft and translucent

Add the broccoli, carrots, and chicken and saute for 10 minutes until almost tender

Add the bok choy, mushrooms, zucchini, and low sodium salt and saute for 5 minutes

Add 1 cup of the water, cover the skillet, and cook for about 10 minutes, until the vegetables are wilted

In a small bowl, dissolve the arrowroot powder in the remaining ½ cup of water, stirring until thoroughly combined

Season at the end with garlic powder, salt and if you like some chilli powder

15. Perfect Eastern Turkey Stir-Fry

Ingredients:
2 tbsp. of coconut oil
2 cloves of garlic (thinly sliced)
1 inch ginger (finely grated)
2-3 green (spring) onions (sliced into long slivers)
1 carrot (coarsely grated)
1 green pepper (sliced into thin, long pieces)
1 turkey breast (cut into bite-sized pieces)
1/4 cup water
2 tbsp. homemade veggie broth
A few drops of toasted sesame oil

Instructions:
Put a pot with a bit of low sodium salt to boil and make sure your rice noodles are handy. Later, when the water has boiled, pop the noodles in and give it a stir.

Heat 2 tbsp. coconut oil in a wok or large pan.

Add the sliced garlic and grated ginger to the wok and stir-fry for 30 seconds.

Add the green onion and stir-fry 1 more minute.

Add the carrot and stir-fry about a minute. You want it just barely cooked, not limp and soggy. Remove the vegetable mixture to a bowl and set aside.

Add another 2/3 tbsp. of coconut oil to the wok.

When the oil is very hot, add the green pepper and stir-fry for 1 minute.

Heat a ½ tbsp. of coconut oil, then add the pieces of turkey breast and stir-fry. I found that the turkey got some color from the previous ingredients that were in the wok. If this doesn't happen, add a tiny amount of soy sauce.

Stir-fry until just done and no more. To check, I like to cut open the biggest piece to make sure it isn't pink in the middle.

Add the sesame oil.

16. Creamy Curry Stir Fry

Ingredients:
2 cooked chicken breasts (small) or 3-4 thighs/legs
3 carrots, chopped
3 sticks celery, chopped
1-2 heads broccoli, chopped
1/2 medium onion, chopped
2 cloves garlic 1/2c coconut milk
1/2c almond or coconut milk
2 tbsp turmeric
2 tbsp curry powder
2 tbsp coconut oil

Instructions:
Put coconut oil in pan and add chopped onion. Cook until onion softens up, add garlic and cook for an additional few minutes.

Next up, add in the carrots, celery, and broccoli. Cook until they have softened a bit (but are not fully cooked).

Shred the cooked chicken up into small pieces for the stir fry and add the coconut milk, other milk, and curry spices.

Stir everything thoroughly, simmer for 5-10 minutes or until everything is cooked to your liking, and serve hot.

Add cauliflower rice (grated cauliflower boiled for 3 minutes)

17. Sexy Turkey Scramble

Ingredients:
1 pound ground turkey
2 medium yellow onions
2 bell peppers (any color)
2 medium squash or zucchini
1 large hand-full of fresh spinach (2-3 ounces)
Spices to taste: I used about 1 tablespoon each of: cumin, chili powder, garlic powder, low sodium salt, and fresh cilantro

Instructions:

Brown the turkey until well cooked in a large skillet or wok over medium high heat.

Remove and add thinly sliced onions, peppers, squash/zucchini to the pan and saute, stirring constantly, until starting to soften.

Return turkey to pan and add fresh spinach.

Spice to taste and continue to cook until spinach is wilted.

Remove and serve with any desired toppings.

18. Turkey Thai Basil

Ingredients:
2 lbs. leftover cooked turkey, cubed or shredded (chicken or shrimp would work too)
3 Tbsp fish sauce
3 Tbsp coconut aminos (or wheat free tamari)
1 Tbsp water
Stevia to taste
1 tsp low sodium salt
1/2 tsp ground white pepper
2 Tbsp coconut oil
4 baby bok choy, leaves pulled apart, hearts halved
1 red bell pepper, sliced
1 yellow bell pepper, sliced
1 large onion, sliced
3 cloves garlic, minced
1 1/2 C lightly pack Thai basil leaves

Instructions:

In a medium bowl, combine turkey with fish sauce, water, low sodium salt and pepper; stir until turkey is thoroughly coated and set aside

Melt coconut oil in large wok or frying pan over medium-high heat

Add bok choy, peppers, onion and garlic and saute until softened, about 8 minutes, stirring frequently

Add contents of set-aside bowl (with the meat) to pan and stir for about 3 minutes until turkey is fully incorporated and heated through

Remove from heat and add Thai basil, stirring until basil wilts

19. Chicken Fennel Stir-Fry

Ingredients:
3 chicken breasts or the meat from 1 whole roasted chicken
2 tablespoons coconut oil
1 onion
1 bulb of fennel
1 teaspoon each of low sodium salt, pepper, garlic powder and basil

Instructions:
Stovetop:

Cut the chicken into bite sized pieces. If chicken is raw, heat butter/coconut oil in large skillet or wok until melted.

Add chicken and cook on medium/high heat until chicken is cooked through. (If chicken is pre-cooked, cook the vegetables first then add chicken)

While cooking, cut the onion into bite sized pieces (1/2 inch) and thinly slice the fennel bulb into thin slivers.

Add all to skillet or wok, add spices and continue sautéing until all are cooked through and fragrant.

This will take approximately 10-12 minutes.

20. Moroccan Madness

Ingredients:
1 chicken breast, chopped into pieces
1/2 tbsp olive oil
1/2 onion, chopped
1 bell pepper, chopped
1 cup diced courgette
2 cloves garlic, minced
1 tsp ginger, minced
1 tsp cumin
1 tsp turmeric
1/2 tsp paprika
1/2 tbsp oregano
1/2 can diced tomatoes
1/2 cup low sodium chicken stock
low sodium salt and pepper

Instructions:

In a pan cook the chicken in the olive oil

Once it's finished cooking, remove from pan and set aside

Add to the pan the bell pepper, onion, courgette, garlic, ginger and all spices, sauté until bell pepper and onion become soft

Add back in the chicken along with the diced tomatoes and chicken stock, let simmer for 10 minutes

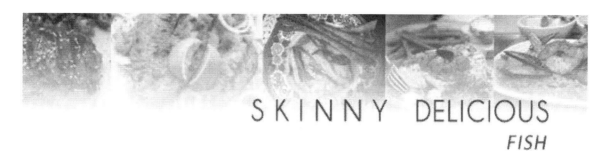

Paleo Epigenetic Fish

21. Thai Baked Fish with Squash Noodles

Ingredients:
1 medium spaghetti squash
Extra virgin olive oil, for drizzling
low sodium salt and pepper
1 tbsp coconut oil
1/2 large onion, finely chopped
1 head broccoli, de-stemmed and cut into florets
2 heads baby bok choy, sliced into 1-inch strips
4 scallions, sliced
1/4 tsp red pepper flakes
1/3 cup cashews, toasted and chopped

For the Sauce:
1 tsp lime juice
1/2-inch piece fresh ginger, peeled and minced
1 clove garlic, minced
1/2 tsp red wine vinegar
3 tbsp almond butter
3 tbsp coconut milk

For the Fish:
2 whole fish fillets…use cod or any good quality white fish

Instructions:
Preheat the oven to 400 degrees F. Place squash in the microwave for 3-4 minutes to soften. Using a sharp knife, cut the squash in half lengthwise. Scoop out the seeds and discard. Place the halves, with the cut side up, on a rimmed baking sheet. Drizzle with olive oil and sprinkle with low sodium salt and pepper. Roast in the oven for 45-50 minutes, until you can poke the squash easily with a fork. Let cool until you can handle it safely. Then scrape the insides with a fork to shred the squash into strands.

While the squash cooks, make the sauce. Combine the lime juice, ginger, garlic, and red wine vinegar in a blender or food processor until smooth. Add the almond butter and coconut milk and blend until completely combined. Adjust the levels of almond butter and coconut milk to reach desired level of creaminess.

Melt the coconut oil in a large pan over medium heat. Add the onion and cook for 5-6 minutes until translucent. Add the broccoli and sauté for 8-10 minutes, until just tender. Then stir in the bok choy and cook for 3-4 minutes until wilted. Lastly add the cooked spaghetti squash into the pan and stir to combine.

To assemble, top the spaghetti squash mixture with the scallions and cilantro. Sprinkle with roasted cashews and drizzle with Thai sauce.

Place the whole fish under the grill at 200 degrees for 25 minutes topped with a tablespoon of olive oil, fresh pressed garlic (one clove) and cayenne pepper to taste.

Finnish off the fish with a squirt of lemon juice to taste.

22. Divine Prawn Mexicana

Ingredients:
1 tbsp extra virgin olive oil
1 tsp chili powder
1 tsp low sodium salt
1 lb. medium shrimp, peeled and deveined
1 avocado, pitted and diced
Shredded lettuce, for serving
Fresh cilantro, for serving
1 lime, cut into wedges

For the tortillas:
6 egg whites
1/4 cup coconut flour
1/4 cup almond milk
1/2 tsp low sodium salt
1/2 tsp cumin
1/4 tsp chili powder

Instructions:

Combine all of the tortilla ingredients together in a small bowl and mix well. Allow the batter to sit for approximately 10 minutes to allow the flour to soak up some of the moisture, and then stir again. The consistency should be similar to crepe batter.

While the batter is resting, heat a skillet to medium-high. Mix together the olive oil, chili powder, and low sodium salt and toss with the shrimp to coat. Cook in the skillet for 1-2 minutes per side, until translucent. Set aside.

Coat the pan with coconut oil spray. Pour about 1/4 cup of batter onto the skillet, turning the pan with your wrist to help it spread out in a thin, even layer. Cook for 1-2 minutes, loosening the sides with a spatula. When the bottom has firmed up, carefully flip over and cook for another 2-3 minutes until lightly browned, then set aside on a plate. Repeat with remaining batter.

Top each tortilla with cooked shrimp, shredded lettuce, avocado, and cilantro. Serve with a lime wedge.

23. Superior Salmon with Lemon and Thyme OR Use any White fish

Ingredients:
32 oz piece of salmon or any fresh white fish
1 lemon, sliced thin
1 tbsp capers
low sodium salt and freshly ground pepper
1 tbsp fresh thyme
Olive oil

Instructions:
Line a rimmed baking sheet with parchment paper and place salmon, skin side down, on the prepared baking sheet.

Season salmon with low sodium salt and pepper. Arrange capers on the salmon, and top with sliced lemon and thyme.

Place baking sheet in a cold oven, then turn heat to 400 degrees F. Bake for 25 minutes. Serve immediately.

24. Spectacular Shrimp Scampi in Spaghetti Sauce

Ingredients:

For the Spaghetti:
1 spaghetti squash
Extra virgin olive oil, for drizzling
low sodium salt and pepper
1 tsp dried oregano
1 tsp dried basil

For the shrimp scampi:
8 oz. shrimp, peeled and deveined
3 tbsp butter
1 tbsp extra virgin olive oil
2 cloves garlic, minced
Pinch of red pepper flakes
low sodium salt and pepper, to taste
1 tbsp fresh parsley, chopped
Juice of 1 lemon
Zest of half a lemon

Instructions:

Preheat the oven to 400 degrees F. Place squash in the microwave for 3-4 minutes to soften. Using a sharp knife, cut the squash in half lengthwise. Scoop out the seeds and discard. Place the halves, with the cut side up, on a rimmed baking sheet.

Drizzle with olive oil and sprinkle with seasonings. Roast in the oven for 45-50 minutes, until you can poke the squash easily with a fork.

Let it cool until you can handle it safely. Then scrape the insides with a fork to shred the squash into strands.

After removing spaghetti squash from the oven, melt the butter and olive oil in a skillet over medium heat.

Add in the garlic and sauté for 2-3 minutes. Then add in the shrimp, low sodium salt, pepper, and a pinch of red pepper flakes.

Cook for 5 minutes, until the shrimp is cooked through. Remove from heat and add in desired amount of cooked spaghetti squash. Toss with lemon juice and zest. Top with parsley.

25. Scrumptious Cod in Delish Sauce

Ingredients:
1 lb. cod fillets
1/3 cup almond flour
1/2 tsp low sodium salt
2-3 tbsp extra virgin olive oil
2 tbsp walnut oil, divided
3/4 cup low sodium chicken stock
3 tbsp lemon juice
1/4 cup capers, drained
2 tbsp fresh parsley, chopped

Instructions:
Stir the almond flour and low sodium salt together in a shallow bowl. Rinse off the fish and pat dry with a paper towel. Dredge the fish in the almond flour mixture to coat.

Heat enough olive oil to coat the bottom of a large skillet over medium-high heat along with one tablespoon walnut oil. Working in batches, add the cod and cook for 2-3 minutes per side to brown. Remove to a plate and set aside.

Add the chicken stock, lemon juice, and capers to the same skillet and scrape any browned bits off the bottom. Simmer to reduce the sauce by almost half. Remove from heat and stir in the remaining tablespoon of walnut oil.

To serve, divide the cod onto plates, drizzle with the sauce, and sprinkle with parsley.

26. Delish Baked dill Salmon

Ingredients:
2 6-oz. salmon fillets
2 zucchini, halved lengthwise and thinly sliced
1/4 red onion, thinly sliced
1 tsp fresh dill, chopped
2 slices lemon
1 tbsp fresh lemon juice
Extra virgin olive oil, for drizzling
low sodium salt and freshly
ground pepper

Instructions:
Preheat the oven to 350 degrees F. Prepare a baking tray

Place half of the zucchini, red onion, dill, and one lemon slice. Drizzle with olive oil and sprinkle with low sodium salt and pepper. Place a salmon fillet on top and drizzle with the lemon juice. Season with low sodium salt and pepper. Repeat with the remaining ingredients.

Bake for 15-20 minutes until the salmon is opaque.

27. Prawn garlic Fried "Rice"

Ingredients:
1 tbsp coconut oil
1 cup white onion, finely chopped
2 cloves garlic, minced
8 oz. prawns peeled and deveined
1 medium carrot, chopped
1/2 cup peas
2 cups cooked cauliflower rice
2 eggs, beaten
Low sodium salt and pepper, to taste

Instructions:
Heat a wok or large pan over medium-high heat. Melt the coconut oil and add the onion and garlic to the pan.

Cook for 3-4 minutes until the onion starts to soften. Add the shrimp and cook for 1 minute.

Add the carrot, peas, and bell pepper to the pan. Cook for 3-4 minutes, and then stir in the cauliflower rice.

Clear a circle in the center of the pan and pour in the beaten eggs. Stir to scramble the eggs and then combine with the other ingredients.

Season with low sodium salt and pepper to taste.

28. Lemon and Thyme Super Salmon

Ingredients:
32 oz piece of salmon
1 lemon, sliced thin
2 tspns lemon juice
Low sodium salt and freshly ground pepper
1 tbsp fresh thyme
Olive oil, for drizzling

Instructions:

Heat a wok or large pan over medium-high heat. Melt the coconut oil and add the onion and garlic to the pan.

Cook for 3-4 minutes until the onion starts to soften. Add the shrimp and cook for 1 minute.

Add the carrot, peas, and bell pepper to the pan. Cook for 3-4 minutes, and then stir in the cauliflower rice.

Clear a circle in the center of the pan and pour in the beaten eggs. Stir to scramble the eggs and then combine with the other ingredients.

Season with low sodium salt and pepper to taste.

29. Delicious Salmon in Herb Crust

Ingredients:
2 salmon fillets (approx. 300g)
1 small onion, peeled and quartered
2 garlic cloves, peeled
1 sprig lemongrass, coarsely chopped
2 cm piece of ginger root, peeled
1 red chili pepper

Instructions:
Line a rimmed baking sheet with parchment paper and place salmon, skin side down, on the prepared baking sheet.

Generously season salmon with low sodium salt and pepper and top with sliced lemon and thyme.

Place baking sheet in a cold oven, then turn heat to 400 degrees F. Bake for 25 minutes.

Add lemon juice and serve immediately.

30. Salmon Mustard Delish

Ingredients:
4 tsp mustard seed
1/2 tsp garlic powder
1/4 tsp low sodium salt
1/4 tsp black pepper
1/4 tsp dried dill
1 1/2 lb salmon

Instructions:
Preheat oven to 200 degrees Celsius. (390 F)

Start by making the herb crust: combine the onion, garlic, lemongrass, ginger in the smallest bowl of a food processor

Process into a coarse paste.

Put the salmon fillets in an oven dish and spread the herb paste on top.

Bake for approx. 12-15 minutes until done, depending on the thickness of your fillets.

Serve with veggies of your choice and enjoy!

31. Sexy Spicy Salmon

Ingredients:

For the Salmon:
4 6 ounce Sockeye Salmon Filets
½ teaspoon of Cinnamon
½ teaspoon of Coriander
½ teaspoon of Cumin
¼ teaspoon of Ground Cloves
¼ teaspoon of Cardamom
low sodium salt to taste
1 Tablespoon of coconut butter

For the Lime Mustard dressing:
¼ cup of olive oil
1 Tablespoon of Lime Juice
2 teaspoons of mustard powder
Pinch of low sodium salt

Instructions:

Preheat the oven to 425°F. Grind all of the spices together with a mortar and pestle until mustard seeds are cracked, most are powder, and everything is well blended.

Spread the mixture over the salmon evenly, and place on a baking pan with a non-stick rack.

Bake for 15 to 20 minutes, until the flesh flakes easily with a fork. If you prefer salmon that is medium-rare, 15 minutes should do the trick.

Enjoy with your favorite sautéed greens, or mixed salad.

32. Mouthwatering Stuffed Salmon

Ingredients:
1 lb wild Alaskan or sockeye salmon, cut into 2 pieces
6 oz raw shrimp, peeled, deveined and chopped
1 large egg
2 tbsp raw onions, chopped
2 tbsp Italian flat leaf parsley, chopped
2 tbsp almond meal (or almond flour)
2 tbsp coconut butter
1 clove garlic, minced
low sodium salt and pepper to taste

Instructions:
For the Salmon:
Preheat oven to 400F
Pat dry the salmon filets with a paper towel.
Combine the cinnamon, coriander, cumin, cloves, and cardamom. Sprinkle evenly over the salmon filet side.
Heat an oven safe skillet (preferably cast iron) to medium high heat. Test the heat by placing a drop of water. It should immediately evaporate.
Add the coconut butter and let it melt.
Place the salmon filet side down and let sear for about 1-2 minutes. Flip and sear on the skin side for 1 minute.
Place the skillet inside the oven, with the skin side down.
Bake at 400F for 6-7 minutes.

For the Lime Mustard Mayo:

Combine dressing, lime juice, low sodium salt, and mustard.

Dip with salmon and enjoy!

33. Spectacular Salmon

Ingredients:

For the salmon:
2 salmon fillets (6oz each)
1 heaping tablespoon coconut flour
2 tablespoons fresh parsley
1 tablespoon olive oil
1 tablespoon mustard powder
low sodium salt and pepper, to taste

For the salad:
2 cups any green leaf salad
¼ red onion, sliced thin
juice of 1 lemon
1 tablespoon white wine vinegar
1 tablespoon olive oil
low sodium salt and pepper, to taste

Instructions:
Preheat oven to 375F.

Mix the chopped raw shrimp, egg, onions, parsley, almond meal, 1tbsp coconut butter, garlic, low sodium salt and pepper. Set aside.

Lightly season the salmon pieces with low sodium salt and pepper. Heat a cast iron pan on high and add the rest of the lard. Pan sear the salmon 1-2 minutes per side.

Move the salmon to an ovenproof dish and top each piece with 2 tbsp (or more!) of the shrimp topping. Lightly brush the top with a little bit of lard and bake in the oven for 15 minutes.

Afterwards, set your oven to broil and cook for about 3 more minutes until the top becomes crispy.

34. Creamy Coconut Salmon

Ingredients:
1 pound wild salmon fillets
¼ tsp low sodium salt
¼ tsp freshly ground black pepper
2 tsp coconut oil
3 cloves fresh garlic (minced)
1 large shallot (minced)
1 lemon (juice and zest)
½ cup unsweetened full-fat coconut milk

Instructions:
Preheat oven to 450 degrees.

Place salmon fillets on a parchment or foil lined baking sheet.

Top your salmon off with olive oil and mustard powder and rub into your salmon.

In a small bowl, mix together your coconut flour, parsley, and low sodium salt and pepper.

Use a spoon to sprinkle on your toppings on your salmon and then your hand to pat into your salmon.

Place in oven for 10-15 minutes or until salmon is cooked to your preference. I cooked mine more on the medium rare side at 12 minutes.

While the salmon is cooking, mix together your salad ingredients.

When salmon is done, place salmon on top of salad and consume.

35. Salmon Dill Bonanza

Ingredients:
1 1/2 pounds wild salmon (I used sockeye)
zest of one lemon (about a tablespoon)
2 tablespoons oil
1 tablespoon chopped, fresh dill
1 lemon
low sodium salt and pepper

Instructions:
Preheat oven to 375°F.

Place salmon in a shallow baking dish and season with low sodium salt and pepper.

Heat coconut oil in a medium saute pan or cast iron skillet over medium heat. Add garlic and shallots and saute until tender and fragrant, 3-5 minutes.

Add lemon zest, lemon juice, and coconut milk, stirring to combine.

Bring to a low boil, then remove from heat.

Pour mixture over salmon. Bake, uncovered, for 10-20 minutes or until salmon flakes easily with a fork.

36. Sexy Shrimp Cocktail

Ingredients:
1 pound uncooked shrimp, peeled, deveined, and thawed if frozen
1 tablespoon olive oil
Low sodium salt and fresh ground pepper to taste
1 cup coconut cream and two tablespoon tomato paste
One teaspoon fresh pressed garlic
lemon wedges

Instructions:
Preheat oven to 400 degrees F.

Oil the bottom of a 9 x 13 baking dish.

Rinse the salmon and pat dry with paper towels. Sprinkle with low sodium salt and pepper and place in the prepared dish.

Mix together the oil (room temperature), lemon zest and dill.

Place about half the mixture on top of the seasoned salmon. You can spread the lemon dill mixture or leave it in dollops like this.

Bake for about 10-15 minutes. The salmon will continue cooking even after you take it out of the oven.

Add the remaining oil/dill/lemon zest mixture on top, add a squeeze of lemon juice.

37. Gambas al Ajillo--Sizzling Garlic Shrimp

Ingredients:
1/2 cup olive oil
10 cloves garlic, peeled and thinly sliced
1 pound raw shrimp, peeled, deveined, and tails removed, defrosted if frozen
Low sodium salt and pepper to taste
1/4 teaspoon paprika
Pinch or two of red pepper flakes, optional

Instructions:
Preheat oven to 425 degrees.

Toss shrimp with oil, low sodium salt and pepper and spread in single layer on rimmed baking sheet.

Roast, turning once, until shrimp is pink and just cooked through (about 5-10 minutes, depending on size of shrimp).

Serve chilled with the blend of coconut cream, tomato paste and pressed garlic…add black pepper and lemon wedges.

38. Garlic Lemon Shrimp Bonanza

Ingredients:
1 lb shrimp, deveined
3-4 cloves of garlic, chopped
1/2 fresh lemon juice
3 tbsp olive oil
1/8 of low sodium salt
Fresh ground pepper (to taste)
1 tbsp fresh parsley, chopped for garnish

Instructions:
Preheat the broiler, if using. Heat the olive oil in a heavy skillet over medium-low heat.

Add the garlic and saute, stirring frequently, for about five minutes, until the garlic is softened but not browned.

Add the shrimp, raise the heat to medium high, and sprinkle with low sodium salt, pepper, paprika, and red pepper.

Cook for three minutes on each side or until the shrimp are completely opaque. Serve hot.

39. Courgette Pesto and Shrimp

Ingredients:

For the Pesto Sauce:
A ton of Basil
Minced Garlic
Pine Nuts
low sodium salt & Pepper

For the Zinguine:
1 Small Zucchini
low sodium salt & Pepper to taste

For the Shrimp:
Shrimp (peeled & de-veined)

Instructions:

Heat pan to medium-high heat.

Add ghee and garlic. Saute for about a minute.

Add shrimp. Saute for about a minute on each side.

Add low sodium salt, pepper and lemon juice. Saute for another minute or so.

Remove from heat and dish onto a plate or bowl.

40. Easy Shrimp Stir Fry

Ingredients:
1lb of wild shrimp
1 Lemon
3 Cloves of garlic, minced
2 Tablespoons of olive oil
1/2 teaspoon of garlic power
1 Dash of red pepper flakes
4 Tablespoons of olive oil

Instructions:
Throw all ingredients in a mini food processor. Pulse until it's a paste that you think looks and smells delicious.

Use a vegetable peeler and peel the courgette right into the pan, then saute.

Stir in pesto sauce and low sodium salt /pepper when the zucchini linguine starts turning transparent.

In another smaller skillet, cook shrimp over medium heat for approximately 3 minutes per side.

41. Delectable Shrimp Scampi

Ingredients:
4 tsp olive oil
1 1/4 pounds med raw shrimp, peeled and deveined (tails left on)
6-8 garlic cloves, minced
1/2 cup low sodium chicken broth
1/4 cup fresh lemon juice
1/4 cup + 1 T minced parsley
1/4 tsp low sodium salt
1/4 tsp freshly ground pepper
4 lemon wedges

Instructions:
Peal shrimp and butterfly them (making a cut in the back and extracting the vein).

Place shrimp in marinade: 2 Tablespoons olive oil, lemon, garlic powder. Marinade anywhere from 15 minutes to hours (the more time, the better)

Heat 2 Tablespoons of oil in pan on medium to high heat.

Add shrimp and cook each side for 2-3 minutes. Drizzle with 1 Tablespoon of olive oil.

Top with low sodium salt, pepper, and red pepper flakes.

42. Citrus Shrimp Delux

Ingredients:
3/4 pounds peeled and deveined medium-large shrimp
1/2 Tbls almond meal
2 Tbls orange juice, fresh squeezed
1/2 Tbls rice vinegar
1 Tbls diced chillies
1 Tbls olive oil
1/2 Tbls fresh ginger, minced
2 garlic cloves, minced

Instructions:

In a large nonstick skillet, heat the oil. Saute the shrimp until just pink, about 2-3 minutes. Add the garlic and cook stirring constantly, about 30 seconds. With a slotted spoon transfer the shrimp to a platter and keep them warm.

In the skillet, combine the broth, lemon juice, 1/4 cup of the parsley, the low sodium salt and pepper; and bring it to a boil. Boil uncovered, until the sauce is reduced by half.

Spoon the sauce over the shrimp. Serve garnished with the lemon wedges and sprinkled with the remaining tablespoon of parsley.

43. Sexy Garlic Shrimp

Ingredients:
4-5 T olive oil
4 garlic cloves, minced
1 t red pepper flakes
1 t smoked paprika
1 lb medium shrimp, peeled and deveined
2 T fresh lime juice
2 Teaspoons jerez sherry
low sodium salt and pepper to taste

Instructions:
Place shrimp in bowl and toss with almond powder.

 Make sure shrimp is evenly coated.

In a small bowl whisk together orange juice, , honey, rice vinegar and chili

Heat olive oil in a large non-stick skillet over medium-high heat. Add ginger and garlic. Stir until garlic becomes fragrant. This will only take 10-15 seconds.

Add shrimp and cook for 3 minutes. Add in sauce and cook for additional 2 minutes. Remove shrimp with a slotted spoon.

Continue stirring sauce for another 2-4 minutes until it thickens. Drizzle over shrimp. Serve on top of baby spinach or fried cauliflower rice.

44. Shrimp Cakes Delux

Ingredients:
2 cups of small prawns
2 eggs
fresh chives
1/2 tsp spicy chili powder
1/2 tsp ground coriander
1/2 tsp garlic powder
shredded coconut
1/2 tbsp coconut flour

Instructions:
In a saute pan over medium heat, warm the olive oil.

Combine all ingredients and blend slightly to get a smoother consistency – but not too much

Make mixture into little cakes – size is your preference

Increase the heat to high, add the shrimp cakes, and saute and turn until the shrimp cake is cooked through – about 3 minutes.

Season with low sodium salt and black pepper.

45. Shrimp Spinach Spectacular

Ingredients:
2 tablespoons olive oil
½ yellow onion – diced
1 cup green beans
2 cloves garlic minced
½ teaspoon chili powder
½ lime – juiced
1 pound raw wild shrimp – thawed, cleaned, and tails removed
1 – 6 oz. bag of baby spinach
low sodium salt and pepper to taste

Instructions:
Chop the shrimp,

Next, mix in the spices, chives, 1 egg and the coconut flour.

Set up 2 bowls, 1 with shredded coconut and the other with the 2nd egg, whisked.

Form cakes of the shrimp mix - cover them with the whisked egg and then with shredded coconut.

Cook them in coconut oil on both sides until brown.

Serve with vegetables of your choice, or fried cauliflower rice.

46. Prawn Salad Boats

Ingredients:
1 lb shrimp, cooked
1 medium tomato, diced
1 cucumber, peeled and diced
3 tablespoons olive oil
One tablespoon coconut cream
Juice of one lemon
1/2 tsp dried dill
1/2 tsp celery seed
1/4 tsp low sodium salt
1/4 tsp pepper
Endive or big lettuce leaf, for serving

Instructions:

In a large sauté pan, heat olive oil over medium heat. Add onion, beans, and sauté until tender – approximately 10 minutes.

Add garlic, lime juice, and chili powder and continue to cook for an additional 5 minutes.

Add spinach and shrimp. Continue to cook for approximately 7-10 more minutes until spinach has wilted and shrimp is done. Place mixture on large lettuce leaves and serve.

47. Cheeky Curry Shrimp

Ingredients:
1 lb raw, peeled, tail on shrimp
2 tsp curry powder
1 tsp garlic powder
1 tsp ground coriander
1/2 tsp ground ginger
low sodium salt and black pepper to taste

Instructions:
In a medium bowl, mix the coconut cream, and lemon juice until combined.

Add the shrimp, tomato, cucumbers, capers, and spices.

Mix until everything is incorporated. Add additional low sodium salt and pepper to taste. Serve in endive leaves.

48. Courgette Shrimp Noodles

Ingredients:
1 pound fresh shrimp, peeled and deveined
4-5 medium courgettes julienned very small, about the size of spaghetti
1 onion, chopped
2 cloves garlic, chopped
1 can diced tomatoes, with liquid (14 oz.)
2 cups fresh spinach
1/2 tsp red chili flake
1 tsp fresh oregano
1 tbsp fresh lemon juice
1 tbsp olive oil

Instructions:
Rinse shrimp under cold water and pat dry with a paper towel.

Place shrimp in a large Ziploc bag.

In a small mixing bowl, curry powder, coriander, garlic powder, ground ginger, low sodium salt, and pepper.

Pour spice mixture over shrimp, seal bag, and toss to evenly coat.

Place shrimp in the fridge and allow to marinate for at least an hour.

Preheat grill to high heat and place all vegetables to grill and crisp for about 15 minutes with 1 tblspn olive oil.

Then grill shrimp about 6 minutes

49. Sexy Shrimp on Sticks

Ingredients:
1/2 lb shrimp, peeled and deveined
1/4 cup coconut milk
1 tsp fish sauce
6 gloves garlic, chopped
1/4 tsp each turmeric, cumin, low sodium salt

Instructions:

Heat olive oil in a large pan over medium heat. Add garlic and spices

Add shrimp and coconut last. Low sodium salt and pepper to taste and serve with a fresh squeeze of lemon.

Serve along side your choice of vegetable or fried cauliflower rice.

50. Delicious Fish Stir Fry

Ingredients:
200 grams any white fish fillet (cut into pieces)
1 Tablespoon Coconut or Apple ciderVinegar
1/2 Teaspoon Ginger and Garlic fresh pressed
1 small onion (quartered)
1/2 Cup Bell Peppers de-seeded and cubed (Red or Yellow).
1/2 Cup Mushrooms (any kind)
2 to 3 stalks of scallions (cut into 1.5 inch length)
low sodium salt to taste
1 Teaspoon Chili powder (Optional)
1 Teaspoon Fish Sauce – low salt
1/2 Tablespoon Extra Virgin Olive Oil

Instructions:

Put a pot with a bit of low sodium salt to boil and make sure your rice noodles are handy. Later, when the water has boiled, pop the noodles in and give it a stir.

Heat 2 tbsp. coconut oil in a wok or large pan.

Add the sliced garlic and grated ginger to the wok and stir-fry for 30 seconds.

Add the green onion and stir-fry 1 more minute.

Add the peppers and stir-fry about a minute. You want it just barely cooked, not limp and soggy. Remove the vegetable mixture to a bowl and set aside.

Add another 2/3 tbsp. of coconut oil to the wok.

When the oil is very hot, add the green pepper and stir-fry for 1 minute.

Heat a ½ tbsp. of coconut oil, then add the pieces of fish and stir-fry. Stir-fry until just done and no more. To check, I like to cut open the biggest piece to make sure it isn't raw in the middle.

Add the sesame oil.

51. Sexy Shrimp with Delish Veggie Stir Fry

Ingredients:
1 1/2 pounds of shrimp
1 tsp. of coconut oil
1/2 cup of thinly sliced onion
1/2 red bell pepper. thinly sliced
1 cup of full fat coconut milk
2 tbsp. fish sauce
1 tbsp curry powder
2 tbsp. of chopped cilantro

Instructions:

In a large bowl mix fish sauce, garlic and ginger.

Heat the olive oil in a wok (or a large nonstick skillet) over medium-high heat.

Once it starts to shimmer add onion and chillies. Stir-fry the onions until they start to brown around the edges, about 2 minutes.

Stir in the bok choy stems and stir-fry for 1 minute.

Add the beaten eggs and cook until it's nearly cooked through about 2 minutes, stirring often.

Stir in bok choy greens, basil and lime juice. And stir-fry for 30 seconds or so, until the greens are wilted. Serve immediately.

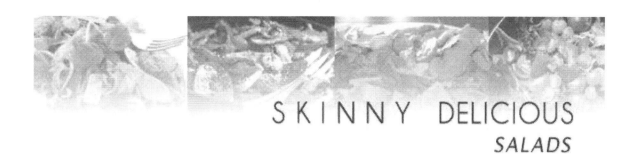

SKINNY DELICIOUS SALADS

Paleo Epigenetic Salads

1. Skinny Delicious Slaw

Ingredients:
1/2 head of cabbage   (mix purple and white)
3 or 4 carrots
1 onion
3 tablespoons walnut oil
1 egg beaten
Stevia and low sdium salt to taste
1 Tbsp. fresh lemon juice
pepper to taste

Instructions:
Grate cabbage, carrots and onion and mix together.

Make dressing by mixing

beaten egg, walnut oil, lemon juice, and seasonings.

Chill and serve.

2. Turkey Eastern Surprise

Ingredients:

For the salad:
2 cups grilled turkey, chopped
6 baby bok choy, grilled & chopped
2 green onions, chopped
1/4 cup cilantro, chopped
1 Tbl sesame seeds

For the dressing:
1 Tbl fresh ginger, chopped
2 Tbl coconut cream
1 Tbl fish sauce
1 Tbl sesame oil
2 Tbl fresh lime juice
1 tsp stevia powder or to taste

Instructions:

Combine all of the salad ingredients until well mixed.

Add all of the ingredients for the dressing into a blender or food processor, and blend until mostly smooth – there may be some small chunks of ginger left, that's ok.

Pour the dressing over the salad and toss lightly until coated.

Garnish with more sesame seeds if desired.

If possible let it sit for an hour in the fridge before serving so the flavors can really meld together.

3. Mediterranean Turkey Delish Salad

Ingredients:
1 roasted turkey (organic, soy-free and pastured is best)
1/2 cup of olive oil
1/4 cup fresh cilantro, chopped
1 head of romaine or butter lettuce
1 red onion, diced
1 lemon, juiced
low sodium salt and pepper as desired

Instructions:
Shred the turkey with your hands or chop up and put it in a big bowl.

Add the oil, red onion, cilantro, lemon, low sodium salt and pepper.

Mix well and serve on a lettuce boat.

4. Skinny Delicious Turkey Divine

Ingredients:
2/3 cup fresh lime juice
1/3 cup fish sauce
Stevia to taste
3/4 cup chicken stock low sodium
1 1/2 pounds ground turkey
1 cup thinly sliced green onions
3/4 cup thinly sliced shallots
3 tablespoons minced lemongrass
1 tablespoon thinly sliced serrano chile
1/2 cup chopped cilantro leaves
1/3 cup chopped mint leaves
low sodium salt
1 head of any lettuce

Instructions:

Whisk together lime juice, fish sauce, honey and chile-garlic sauce. Set aside.

Warm chicken stock in a medium heavy-bottomed pot over medium heat until simmering. Add ground turkey and simmer until cooked through. As the turkey is cooking, stir occasionally to break up the meat. This should take 6 to 8 minutes.

Add green onion, shallot, lemongrass and chiles, stirring to combine. Continue cooking until shallots turn translucent, stirring occasionally (about 4 minutes). Remove from the heat and drain off any liquid in the pot

Stir in lime juice-fish sauce mixture, cilantro and mint. Season to taste with low sodium salt (not much is needed if any).

Transfer mixture to a large bowl and serve beside a pile of lettuce leaves. Using a spoon, scoop on to the lettuce leaves and enjoy!

5. Chicken Basil Avo Salad

Ingredients:
2 boneless, skinless chicken breasts (organic, cooked and shredded)
1/2 cup fresh basil leaves, stems removed
1 cup sliced cherry tomatoes
2 small or 1 large ripe avocado, pits and skin removed
2 Tbsp. extra virgin olive oil
1/2 tsp. low sodium salt (or more to taste)
1/8 tsp. ground black pepper (or more to taste)

Instructions:
Place the cooked shredded chicken in a medium sized mixing bowl.

Place the basil, avocado, olive oil, low sodium salt and ground black pepper in a food processor and blend until smooth. You may need to scrape the sides a couple times to incorporate.

Pour the avocado and basil mixture into the mixing bowl with the shredded chicken and tomatoes and toss well to coat.

Taste and add additional low sodium salt and ground black pepper if desired. Keep in the fridge until ready to serve.

6. Skinny Chicken salad

Ingredients:

Salad:
1 small head (or 4 cups) savoy cabbage, finely shredded –
1 cup carrot, julienned
1/4 cup scallions, trimmed and julienned
1/4 cup radishes, julienned
1/4 cup fresh cilantro, chopped
1/4 cup fresh mint, chopped
2 cups cooked organic chicken

Vinaigrette:
2 tablespoons coconut or rice vinegar
2 tablespoons sesame oil (use unrefined or cold-pressed)
juice of 1/2 a lime
1 chipotle pepper - optional
1 clove garlic, crushed
1 teaspoon fresh ginger, grated

Instructions:

Salad – Combine cabbage, carrots, scallions and radishes. Top with chicken, cilantro and mint and set aside.

Vinaigrette –Combine the vinaigrette ingredients. Taste to see if it needs any adjustments. If it is too spicy, you can add more lime juice to counteract it.

Drizzle salad with vinaigrette & enjoy.

7. Turkey Taco Salad

Ingredients:
1/2 lbs (ish) leftover turkey, cooked and chopped
1 1/2 Tbsp taco seasoning (recipe follows)
1 tblsp. coconut or olive oil and 1 tblsp rice vinegar
1/4 c. water
Shredded lettuce

Optional Toppings - sliced olives, tomatoes, red onion, avocado, bell peppers, crushed sweet potato chips

Taco Seasoning:
Mix together, 4 Tbsp. chili powder, 1 tsp each garlic powder, onion powder, and oregano, 2 tsp each paprika and cumin, 4 tsp low sodium salt, and 1/8-1/4 tsp red pepper flakes.

Instructions:
In a skillet, heat 1 teaspoon oil and add in chicken - I like to fry it for a minute to give some extra flavor. Add in water and taco seasoning, let simmer until liquid is gone.

Meanwhile, shred, chop, and dice all your toppings.

Assemble, lettuce, optional toppings, chicken, leftover oil and vinegar dressing, and crushed chips.

8. Cheeky Turkey Salad

Ingredients:
For the Turkey:
1 lb boneless turkey breasts
1 tbsp olive oil
low sodium salt and pepper, to taste

For the Salsa:
1 large tomato, quartered
1/2 red onion, cut into large chunks
1 garlic clove, peeled
1 small bunch of cilantro leaves
Juice of 1 lime
low sodium salt and pepper, to taste

Instructions:
Preheat oven to 375 F.

Bake turkey breasts dipped in olive oil on a baking sheet for 35 to 40 minutes, until no longer pink in the center.

While baking, add all salsa ingredients to a food processor and pulse using the chopping blade until finely chopped. Transfer the salsa to a large bowl and clean out the food processor. You will be using it to shred the turkey.

(If you don't have a food processor, just dice the tomato, onion, pepper, cilantro and garlic and add to a bowl with the lime juice, low sodium salt and pepper).

Remove turkey from the oven and allow to cool. Once cool enough to handle, cut each breast into three or four smaller pieces and add to the food processor. Pulse using the chopping blade until shredded.

Add turkey to bowl with salsa and mix well with a fork.

Refrigerate for at least two hours until turkey salad is chilled.

9. Macadamia Chicken Salad

Ingredients:
1lb organic chicken breast
1tsp macadamia nut oil, or oil of choice
few pinches of low sodium salt and pepper
1/2 cup macadamia nuts, chopped
1/2 cup diced celery
2 tbsp julienned basil
1 tablespoon olive oil and 2 teaspoons rice vinegar
1 tbsp lemon juice

Instructions:
Preheat oven to 350. Place chicken breasts on sheet tray, drizzle will oil and a pinch of low sodium salt and pepper. Bake for about 35 minutes until cooked through. Remove from oven and let cool.

In a large bowl shred chicken. Add nuts, celery, basil, dressing, and a pinch of low sodium salt and pepper. Gently stir until combined. Eat!

10. Rosy Chicken Supreme Salad

Ingredients:
For the chicken:
450g chicken mince, free range of course
1 long red chili, finely chopped with the seeds
2 garlic cloves, finely chopped
Little nob of fresh ginger, peeled and finely chopped
1 stem lemon grass, pale section only, finely chopped
1/2 bunch of coriander stems washed and finely chopped (I don't waste anything, save the leaves for the salad)
2 1/2 tbsp fish sauce
1/2 lime rind grated
1/2 lime, juiced
A pinch of low sodium salt
Coconut oil for frying (about 3 tablespoons)

For the salad:
1/4 red cabbage, thinly sliced
1 large carrot, peeled and grated
1/2 Spanish onion, thinly sliced
2 tbsp green spring onion, chopped
1/2 bunch of fresh coriander leaves (saved from the stems used in the chicken)
A handful of fresh mint or Thai basil if available
1/2 cup crashed roasted cashews or some sesame seeds

For the dressing:
2 tbsp olive oil
3 tbsp lime juice
1 tbsp fish sauce
1 small red chili, finely chopped

Instructions:
Once you've prepared all your ingredients for the chicken, heat 1 tbsp of coconut oil in a large frying pan or a wok to high.

Throw in lemongrass, chili, garlic, coriander stems and ginger and stir fry for about a minute until fragrant.

Add chicken mince and lime zest. Stir and break apart the mince with a wooden mixing spoon until separated into small chunks (this might take a while as chicken mince is quite sticky).

The meat will now be changing to white colour.

Add fish sauce and lime juice. Stir through and cook for a further few minutes. Total cooking time for the chicken should be about 10 minutes.

Prepare the salad base by mixing together sliced red cabbage, onion grated carrot, and fresh herbs.

Mix all dressing ingredients and toss through the salad.

Serve cooked chicken mince on top of the dressed salad and topped with roasted cashews, dried shallots, coconut flakes and extra fresh herbs.

11. Turkey Sprouts Salad

Ingredients:
1/2 pound of brussels sprouts (2-ish cups once sliced)
1/2 cup chopped almonds
2 turkey breasts, chopped
1/2 white onion, finely diced

Vinaigrette:
2 TBSP Apple Cider Vinegar
1 TBSP quality mustard powder
1 TBSP avocado oil
Stevia to taste
1/2 tsp low sodium salt
few grinds of black pepper

Instructions:
Cut the brussels sprouts in half and thinly slice. Chop the half cup of almonds. Finely dice the white onion. Scallions would work too if you prefer a more mild onion flavor… though the white did not overpower.

Remove the breasts and chop into bite-sized pieces. Combine all of these ingredients into a large bowl and gently toss the Brussels sprouts salad.

Whipping up the vinaigrette takes seconds. Add all ingredients to a small bowl and whisk until smooth. Pour over the Brussels sprouts salad and toss to bring together.

12. Delicious Chicken Salad

Ingredients:
Cooked and chopped chicken breast
Chopped almonds
Mashed avocado
Lots of low sodium salt and pepper
Any lettuce leaves of choice

Instructions:
Mix the first six ingredients together in a bowl, season with low sodium salt and pepper, and then spoon onto lettuce leaves. Roll up and enjoy!

13. Avocado Tuna Salad

Ingredients:
2 tins high quality albacore tuna
1 avocado
1/4 of an onion, chopped
juice of 1/2 a lime
2 Tbsp cilantro (or sub basil if you prefer)
some low sodium salt and pepper, to taste

Instructions:
Shred the tuna.

Add all of the other ingredients and mix.

14. Classic Tuna Salad

Ingredients:
2 large grilled tuna steaks
2 tablespoons olive oil
.5 cup onion, chopped (I like red, scallions are also good)
2-3 stalks celery, chopped (or .5 cup)
.5 – .75 cup pecans, chopped (optional)
.5 – 1 tsp low sodium salt
.5 tsp Lemon Garlic pepper
.5 – 1 Tbsp lemon juice

Instructions:
Grill the tuna steaks medium rare with garlic powder and black pepper to taste

Then do a bunch of chopping. Onions, celery, and pecans.

Combine all of these ingredients in the bowl with your cubed tuna and then start adding the dressing of oil and lemon juice seasoned.

You want enough to cover all the ingredients and make them moist, but not overly runny or dry.

It tastes great served right away, but even better after it sits in the fridge for a day.

15. Artichoke Tuna Delight

Ingredients:
1.5 cups diced grilled tuna
¼ cup finely diced red onion
1 small carrot julienned and cut into small pieces (or ½ a diced red bell pepper)
4-5 artichoke hearts (I used canned in water) diced
2 tablespoons capers
low sodium salt and pepper to taste.
6 Radicchio leaves

Instructions:
Place all ingredients, except the radicchio leaves in a large bowl and combine.

Place a scoop if salad into each Radicchio cup and serve.

Store salad in an air tight container in the fridge.

16. Tasty Tuna Stuffed Tomato

Ingredients:
2 large tomatoes
Lettuce leaves (optional)
2 (5 or 6 oz.) cans wild albacore tuna
6 Tbsp. olive oil and 1 tablespoon rice vinegar
1 stalk celery, chopped
1/2 small onion, chopped
1/4 tsp. low sodium salt
1/4 tsp. ground black pepper

Instructions:
Wash and dry the tomatoes and remove any stem. You can either slice off the top part of the tomatoes and hollow them out, or cut each tomato into wedges, making sure to only cut down to about 1/2 inch before you get to the bottom of the tomato.

Arrange the tomatoes on a plate on top of lettuce leaves (optional).

Combine the remaining ingredients in a mixing bowl and add additional low sodium salt and/or pepper if desired. Spoon into the tomatoes and serve.

17. Advanced Avocado Tuna Salad

Ingredients:
1 avocado
1 lemon, juiced, to taste
1 tablespoon chopped onion, to taste
1 cup chopped tomatoes
5 ounces cooked or canned wild tuna
low sodium salt and pepper to taste

Instructions:
Cut the avocado in half and scoop the middle of both avocado halves into a bowl, leaving a shell of avocado flesh about 1/4-inch thick on each half.

Add lemon juice and onion to the avocado in the bowl and mash together.

Add tuna, low sodium salt and pepper, and stir to combine. Taste and adjust if needed.

Fill avocado shells with tuna salad and serve.

18. Sexy Italian Tuna Salad

Ingredients:
10 sun-dried tomatoes
2 (5 oz) can of tuna
1-2 ribs of celery, diced finely
2 Tablespoons of extra virgin olive oil
1 cloves garlic, minced
3 Tablespoons finely chopped parsley
1/2 Tablespoon lemon juice
low sodium salt and pepper to taste

Instructions:
Prepare the sun-dried tomatoes by softening them in warm water for 30 minutes until soft. Then, pat the tomatoes dry and chop finely.

Flake the tuna.

Mix the tuna together with the chopped tomatoes, celery, extra virgin olive oil, garlic, parsley, and lemon juice. Add low sodium salt and pepper to taste.

If not serving immediately, mix with extra olive oil just before serving.

Optional: Make cucumber boats with them.

19. Divine Chicken or Turkey and Baby Bok Choy Salad

Ingredients:

For the salad:
2 cups grilled chicken or turkey, chopped
6 baby bok choy, grilled & chopped
2 green onions, chopped
1/4 cup cilantro, chopped
1 Tbl sesame seeds

For the dressing:
1 Tbl fresh ginger, chopped
2 Tbl coconut cream
1 Tbl sesame oil
2 Tbl fresh lime juice
1 tsp stevia powder

Instructions:

Combine all of the salad ingredients until well mixed.

Add all of the ingredients for the dressing into a blender or food processor, and blend until mostly smooth

Pour the dressing over the salad and toss lightly until coated.

Garnish with more sesame seeds if desired.

20. Mediterranean Medley Salad

Ingredients:
1 roasted chicken (organic, soy-free and pastured is best).. or turkey or ostrich steak

Dressing:
1/2 cup of olive oil, ¼ cup applecider vinegar and
    garlick powder and chilli powder to taste
1/4 cup fresh cilantro, chopped
1 head of romaine or butter lettuce
1 red onion, diced
1 lemon, juiced
low sodium salt and pepper as desired

Instructions:
Shred the chicken/turkey etc or chop up and put it in a big bowl.

Add the dressing…also red onion, cilantro, lemon, low sodium salt and pepper.

Mix well and serve on a lettuce boat.

21. Spicy Eastern Salad

Ingredients:
2/3 cup fresh lime juice
1/3 cup fish sauce(optional)
Stevia to taste
3/4 cup low sodium chicken stock (preferably homemade)
1 1/2 pounds ground chicken or turkey
1 cup thinly sliced green onions
3/4 cup thinly sliced shallots
3 tablespoons minced lemongrass
1 tablespoon thinly sliced serrano or other chile - optional
1/2 cup chopped cilantro leaves
1/3 cup chopped mint leaves
low sodium salt
1 head of butter lettuce or other green leaves

Instructions:

Whisk together lime juice, fish sauce (optional – try low sodium version)..stevia and Set aside.

Warm chicken stock in a medium heavy-bottomed pot over medium heat until simmering.

Add ground chicken and simmer until cooked through. As the chicken is cooking, stir occasionally to break up the meat. This should take 6 to 8 minutes.

Add green onion, shallot, lemongrass and chiles, stirring to combine. Continue cooking until shallots turn translucent, stirring occasionally (about 4 minutes).

Remove from the heat and drain off any liquid in the pot. I do this by clamping the lid on, then cracking it just a hair. I turn the entire pot over the sink and let the liquid drain out.

Stir in lime juice-fish sauce mixture, cilantro and mint. Season to taste with low sodium salt (not much is needed if any).

Transfer mixture to a large bowl and serve beside a pile of lettuce leaves. Using a slotted spoon, scoop on to the lettuce leaves and enjoy!

22. Basil Avocado Bonanza Salad

Ingredients:
2 boneless, skinless chicken or turkey breasts (cooked and shredded)
1/2 cup fresh basil leaves, stems removed
2 small or 1 large ripe avocado, pits and skin removed
2 Tbsp. extra virgin olive oil
1/2 tsp. low sodium salt (or more to taste)
1/8 tsp. ground black pepper (or more to taste)

Instructions:
Place the cooked shredded chicken in a medium sized mixing bowl.

Place the basil, avocado, olive oil, low sodium salt and ground black pepper in a food processor and blend until smooth.

Pour the avocado and basil mixture into the mixing bowl with the shredded chicken and toss well to coat.

Taste and add additional low sodium salt and ground black pepper if desired. Keep in the fridge until ready to serve.

23. Chinese Divine Salad

Ingredients:

Salad :
1 small head (or 4 cups) savoy cabbage, finely shredded –
1 cup carrot, julienned (about 1 large carrot)
1/4 cup scallions, trimmed and julienned (about 3 scallions)
1/4 cup radishes, julienned
1/4 cup fresh cilantro, chopped
1/4 cup fresh mint, chopped
2 cups cooked chicken or turkey

Vinaigrette:
2 tablespoons coconut or rice vinegar
Low sodium salt to taste
2 tablespoons sesame oil
1 chipotle pepper
1/2 teaspoon chilli flakes
1 clove garlic, crushed
1 teaspoon fresh ginger, grated
Stevia to taste

Instructions:

Salad – Combine cabbage, carrots, scallions and radishes. Top with chicken, cilantro and mint and set aside.

Vinaigrette –Combine the vinaigrette ingredients. Taste to see if it needs any adjustments. If it is too spicy, you can add more lime juice to counteract it.

Drizzle salad with vinaigrette & enjoy

24. Divinely Delish Salad Surprise

Ingredients:
1/2 lbs (ish) leftover chicken, turkey or boiled egg cooked and chopped
1 tsp. coconut or olive oil
1/4 c. water
Shredded lettuce
Optional Toppings - sliced olives, tomatoes, red onion, avocado, bell peppers
Non-optional Toppings - crushed sweet potato chips

Divine Dressing:
Mix together, 4 Tbsp. chili powder, 1 tsp each garlic powder, onion powder, and oregano, 2 tsp each paprika and cumin, 4 tsp low sodium salt, and 1/8-1/4 tsp red pepper flakes. Add 1 cup olive oil and half cup rice vinegar

Instructions:
Then, in a skillet, heat the oil and add in chicken etc –. Add in water let simmer until liquid is gone.

Meanwhile, shred, chop, and dice all your toppings.

Assemble, lettuce, optional toppings, chicken, dressing, and crushed chips.

Add Divine Dressing.

25. Avocado Salad with Cilantro and Lime

Ingredients:
Turkey Breast chopped
Two avocados, diced
2/3 green cabbage, chopped
5 green onions (scallions), white and pale green parts, minced
Juice of 2 limes
Two handfuls of fresh cilantro, chopped
low sodium salt to taste
One large English Cucumber

Instructions:
Mix all ingredients except cucumber -slice it thinly and use it as a base for the salad. For "party style", slice 1-2 inch sections, scoop out the center with a grapefruit spoon, and fill the cucumber "cups" with the salad.

Divine Dressing:
Mix together, 4 Tbsp. chili powder, 1 tsp each garlic powder, onion powder, and oregano, 2 tsp each paprika and cumin, 4 tsp low sodium salt, and 1/8-1/4 tsp red pepper flakes. Add 1 cup olive oil and half cup rice vinegar.

26. Mexican Medley Salad

Ingredients:
For the Chicken or turkey:
1 lb boneless chicken/turkey breasts
1 tbsp olive oil
low sodium salt and pepper, to taste

For the Salsa:
1 large tomato, quartered
1/2 red onion, cut into large chunks
1 jalapeno pepper, stem and seeds removed and halved
1 garlic clove, peeled
1 small bunch of cilantro leaves
Juice of 1 lime
low sodium salt and pepper, to taste

Instructions:
Preheat oven to 375 F.

Brush chicken breasts on both sides with olive oil and sprinkle with low sodium salt and pepper. Bake on a baking sheet for 35 to 40 minutes, until no longer pink in the center.

While chicken is baking, add all salsa ingredients to a food processor and pulse using the chopping blade until finely chopped.

Transfer the salsa to a large bowl and clean out the food processor. You will be using it to shred the chicken.

Remove chicken from the oven and allow to cool. Once cool enough to handle, cut each breast into three or four smaller pieces and add to the food processor. Pulse using the chopping blade until shredded.

Add chicken to bowl with salsa and mix well with a fork.

Refrigerate for at least two hours until chicken salad is chilled.

27. Macadamia Nut Chicken/Turkey Salad

Ingredients:
1lb chicken/turkey breast
1tsp macadamia nut oil, or oil of choice
few pinches of low sodium salt and pepper
1/2 cup macadamia nuts, chopped
1/2 cup diced celery
3 tbsp divine dressing
2 tbsp julienned basil
1 tbsp lemon juice

Instructions:
Preheat oven to 350. Place chicken breasts on sheet tray, drizzle will oil and a pinch of low sodium salt and pepper.

Bake for about 35 minutes until cooked through. Remove from oven and let cool.

In a large bowl shred chicken. Add nuts, celery, basil, mayo, lemon juice, and a pinch of low sodium salt and pepper. Gently stir until combined. Eat!

Divine Dressing:
Mix together, 4 Tbsp. chili powder, 1 tsp each garlic powder, onion powder, and oregano, 2 tsp each paprika and cumin, 4 tsp low sodium salt, and 1/8-1/4 tsp red pepper flakes. Add 1 cup olive oil and half cup rice vinegar.

28. Red Cabbage Bonanza Salad

Ingredients:
For the chicken or turkey:
450g chicken/turkey mince, free range of course
1 long red chili, finely chopped with the seeds
2 garlic cloves, finely chopped
Little nob of fresh ginger, peeled and finely chopped
1 stem lemon grass, pale section only, finely chopped
1/2 bunch of coriander stems washed and finely chopped (I don't waste anything, save the leaves for the salad)
1 tbs low sodium salt
1 tbsp coconut aminos
1/2 lime rind grated
1/2 lime, juiced
A pinch of low sodium salt
Coconut oil for frying (about 3 tablespoons)

For the salad:
1/4 red cabbage, thinly sliced
1 large carrot, peeled and grated
1/2 Spanish onion, thinly sliced
2 tbsp green spring onion, chopped
1/2 bunch of fresh coriander leaves (saved from the stems used in the chicken)
A handful of fresh mint or Thai basil if available
1/2 cup crashed roasted cashews or some seasame seeds
1/2 cup dried fried shallots (optional for garnish)
2 tbsp toasted coconut flakes (optional for garnish)

For the dressing:
2 tbsp olive oil
3 tbsp lime juice
1 small red chili, finely chopped (you can leave it out if you like it mild)

Instructions:
Once you've prepared all your ingredients for the chicken, heat 1 tbsp of coconut oil in a large frying pan or a wok to high. Throw in lemongrass, chili, garlic, coriander stems and ginger and stir fry for about a minute until fragrant.

Add chicken mince and lime zest. Stir and break apart the mince with a wooden mixing spoon until separated into small

The meat will now be changing to white colour. Add lime juice. Stir through and cook for a further few minutes. Total cooking time for the chicken should be about 10 minutes.

Prepare the salad base by mixing together sliced red cabbage, onion grated carrot, and fresh herbs.

Mix all dressing ingredients and toss through the salad.

Serve cooked chicken mince on top of the dressed salad and topped with roasted cashews, dried shallots, coconut flakes and extra fresh herbs.

29. Spectacular Sprouts Salad

Ingredients:
1/2 pound of mixed sprouts (2-ish cups once sliced)
1/2 Granny Smith apple
1/2 cup chopped almonds
2 chicken breasts, chopped
1/2 white onion, finely diced

Vinaigrette:
2 TBSP Apple Cider Vinegar
1 TBSP quality brown mustard
1 TBSP avocado oil
Stevia to taste
1/2 tsp low sodium salt
few grinds of black pepper

Instructions:
Cut Granny Smith apple, slicing into matchsticks.

Chop the half cup of almonds. Finely dice the white onion. Scallions would work too if you prefer a more mild onion flavor… though the white did not overpower.

Remove the breasts and chop into bite-sized pieces. Combine all of these ingredients into a large bowl and gently toss the sprouts into the salad.

Whipping up the vinaigrette takes seconds. Add all ingredients to a small bowl and whisk until smooth. Pour over the sprouts salad and toss to bring together.

30. Avocado Egg Salad

Ingredients:
Cooked and chopped organic eggs x 3
Chopped almonds
Mashed avocado
low sodium salt and pepper
Any lettuce leaves

Instructions:
Mix the ingredients together in a bowl, season with low sodium salt and pepper, and then spoon onto lettuce leaves. Roll up and enjoy!

31. Avocado Divine Salad

Ingredients:
1 kilo boneless, skinless chicken or turkey breasts (2 or 3)
1 avocado
1/4 of an onion, chopped
juice of one lime and one lemon
2 Tbsp cilantro (or sub basil if you prefer)
some low sodium salt and pepper, to taste
One bag mixed lettuce leaves
One tablespoon olive oil

Instructions:
Cook chicken breast until done, let cool, and then shred. Add all of the other ingredients and mix.

32. Classic Waldorf Salad

Ingredients:
half whole cooked chicken or turkey (~2lbs)
half cup apple, peeled and chopped (optional)
half cup onion, chopped (I like red, scallions are also good)
2-3 stalks celery, chopped (or .5 cup)
half cup pecans, chopped (optional)
half tsp low sodium salt
half tsp Lemon Garlic
pepper
1 Tbsp lemon juice

Divine Dressing:
Mix together, 4 Tbsp. chili powder, 1 tsp each garlic powder, onion powder, and oregano, 2 tsp each paprika and cumin, 4 tsp low sodium salt, and 1/8-1/4 tsp red pepper flakes. Add 1 cup olive oil and half cup rice vinegar

Instructions:
First cook up a whole chicken. You can buy a rotisserie chicken, or do what I do, throw a chicken in the crockpot, sprinkle it with cumin, low sodium salt & pepper and let it cook for about 4-6 hours on low.

After the chicken is cooked and cooled, de-bone and shred the meat (white and dark) and put it in a large mixing bowl. I usually use about half of my 3-4lb chicken.

Then do a bunch of chopping. Peel your apple, then chop your apple, onions, celery, and pecans.

Combine all of these ingredients in the bowl with your chicken and then start adding the dressing. You want enough to cover all the ingredients and make them moist, but not overly runny or dry.

Add the low sodium salt and pepper, and lemon juice Stir well to combine. Add dressing.

33. Artichoke Heart & Turkey Salad Radicchio Cups

Ingredients:
1.5 cups diced cooked turkey
¼ cup finely diced red onion
1 small carrot julienned and cut into small pieces (or ½ a diced red bell pepper)
4-5 artichoke hearts (I used canned in water) dicedlow sodium salt and pepper to taste.
6 Radicchio leaves

Instructions:
Place all ingredients, except the radicchio leaves in a large bowl and combine.

Place a scoop if salad into each Radicchio cup and serve.

Store salad in an air tight container in the fridge.

Divine Dressing:
Mix together, 4 Tbsp. chili powder, 1 tsp each garlic powder, onion powder, and oregano, 2 tsp each paprika and cumin, 4 tsp low sodium salt, and 1/8-1/4 tsp red pepper flakes. Add 1 cup olive oil and half cup rice vinegar.

34. Tempting Tuna Stuffed Tomato

Ingredients:
2 large tomatoes
Lettuce leaves (optional)
2 (5 or 6 oz.) cans wild albacore tuna
1 stalk celery, chopped
1/2 small onion, chopped
1/4 tsp. low sodium salt
1/4 tsp. ground black pepper

Instructions:
Wash and dry the tomatoes and remove any stem.

Arrange the tomatoes on a plate on top of lettuce leaves (optional).

Combine the remaining ingredients in a mixing bowl and add additional low sodium salt and/or pepper if desired.

Spoon into the tomatoes and serve.

35. Incredibly Delish Avocado Tuna Salad

Ingredients:
1 avocado
1 lemon, juiced, to taste
1 tablespoon chopped onion, to taste
5 ounces cooked or canned wild tuna
low sodium salt and pepper to taste

Instructions:
Cut the avocado in half and scoop the middle of both avocado halves into a bowl, leaving a shell of avocado flesh about 1/4-inch thick on each half.

Add lemon juice and onion to the avocado in the bowl and mash together. Add tuna, low sodium salt and pepper, and stir to combine. Taste and adjust if needed.

Fill avocado shells with tuna salad and serve.

36. Italian Tuna Bonanza Salad

Ingredients:
10 sun-dried tomatoes
2 (5 oz) can of tuna
1-2 ribs of celery, diced finely
2 Tablespoons of extra virgin olive oil
1 cloves garlic, minced
3 Tablespoons finely chopped parsley
1/2 Tablespoon lemon juice
low sodium salt and pepper to taste

Instructions:

Prepare the sun-dried tomatoes by softening them in warm water for 30 minutes until soft. Then, pat the tomatoes dry and chop finely.

Flake the tuna. and mix the tuna together with the chopped tomatoes, celery, extra virgin olive oil, garlic, parsley, and lemon juice. Add low sodium salt and pepper to taste.

If not serving immediately, mix with extra olive oil just before serving.

Optional: Make cucumber boats with them.

37. Asian Aspiration Salad

Ingredients:
1 red bell pepper, sliced
1 large carrot, cut into matchsticks
1 cucumber, halved lengthwise and sliced

Optional:
fresh ginger juice and rice vinegar
2 boiled eggs

Instructions:
Mix ingredients and Serve.

38. Tasty Carrot Salad

Ingredients:
5 carrots, medium
1 tbs. whole black mustard seeds
1/4 tsp. low sodium salt
2 tsp. lemon juice
2 tbs. olive oil
Add 1 Grated egg on top

Instructions:
Trim and peel and grate carrots. In a bowl, toss with low sodium salt and set aside.

In a small heavy pan over medium heat, heat oil.

When very hot, add mustard seeds. As soon as the seeds begin to pop, in a few seconds, pour oil and seeds over carrots.

Add lemon juice and toss. Serve at room temperature or cold.

Add Grated egg.

39. Creamy Carrot Salad

Ingredients:
1 pound carrots - shredded
20 ounces crushed pineapple -- drained
8 ounces Coconut milk
3/4 cup flaked coconut
Stevia to taste
Shredded turkey one breast

Instructions:
Combine all ingredients, tossing well. Cover and chill.

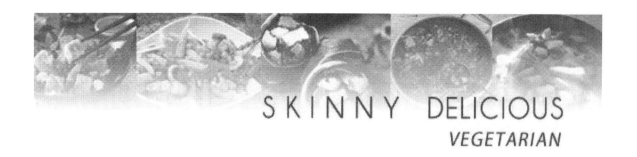

Paleo Epigenetic Pure Vegetables

1. Vegetarian Curry with Squash

Ingredients:
1 tbsp coconut oil
2 cups mixed raw nuts.
1 medium yellow onion, diced
1 tsp low sodium salt
1 green bell pepper, thinly sliced
4 cloves garlic, minced
1-inch piece fresh ginger, peeled and minced
1 14-oz. can coconut milk
1 large acorn squash, peeled, seeded, and cut into 1-inch cubes
2 tsp lime juice
One teaspoon curry powder (mild or hot)
1/4 cup cilantro, chopped
Cauliflower rice, for serving

Instructions:
Melt the coconut oil in a large pan over medium heat. Add the onion and cook for 5-6 minutes, stirring occasionally. Add the bell pepper, garlic, ginger, and low sodium salt and stir to combine. Cook for an additional minute.

Add the curry powder to the pan and cook for about a minute, stirring to coat the other ingredients. Add in the coconut milk and bring to a simmer. Stir in the squash.

Simmer, stirring occasionally, for 15-20 minutes until the squash is fork-tender. Remove the pan from the heat and stir in the lime juice. Taste and adjust low sodium salt and lime juice as necessary. Sprinkle with cilantro to serve.

Roast the nuts under the grill until crisp and sprinkle over the top of the curry.

Serve with Cauliflower rice!

2. Saucy Gratin with Creamy Cauliflower Bonanza

Ingredients:
1 medium butternut squash, peeled, seeded, and diced
1 large sweet potato, peeled and thinly sliced
6 cups fresh spinach
1 tbsp extra virgin olive oil
2 large shallots, diced
4 cloves garlic, chopped
low sodium salt and pepper, to taste
Pinch of nutmeg

For the sauce:
1/2 head of cauliflower, cut into florets
1 cup almond milk
1/2 cup low sodium chicken stock
1/2 tsp low sodium salt
1/2 tsp freshly ground pepper
1/4 tsp nutmeg

Instructions:
Preheat the oven to 375 degrees F. To make the cream sauce, place a couple inches of water in a large pot. Once the water is boiling, place steamer insert and then cauliflower florets into the pot and cover. Steam for 12-14 minutes, until completely tender.

Drain and return cauliflower to the pot. Add the almond milk, stock, nutmeg, low sodium salt, and pepper to the pot. Use an immersion blender or food processor to combine the ingredients until smooth. Set aside.

Meanwhile, bring a separate pot of water to a boil. Add the butternut squash and cook for 4 minutes. Drain and set aside.

Heat the oil in a small pan over medium heat. Add the shallots and garlic and cook for 4-5 minutes until soft. Stir in the spinach to wilt. Season with low sodium salt and pepper.

To assemble, grease a large baking dish with coconut oil spray. Spoon a thin layer of the cream sauce over the bottom of the pan.

Arrange a layer of half of the butternut squash. Top with half of the spinach mixture, and then all of the sliced sweet potato.

Drizzle with the cream sauce. Add the remaining half of the spinach, followed by the rest of the butternut squash. Drizzle the rest of the cream sauce over the top.

Sprinkle with low sodium salt, pepper, and nutmeg. Bake for 50-60 minutes until browned. Allow to cool for 10 minutes.

3. Egg Bok Choy and Basil Stir-Fry

Ingredients:
1 garlic clove, minced
3 organic eggs
2 tablespoons olive oil
1 small onion, finely chopped
1-inch piece fresh ginger, chopped
2 red chiles, thinly sliced crosswise
1 cup thinly sliced bok choy stems
1 cup thinly sliced bok choy greens
handful fresh basil leaves, chopped
juice of 1 lime

Instructions:

In a large bowl mix garlic and ginger.

Heat the olive oil in a wok (or a large nonstick skillet) over medium-high heat.

Once it starts to shimmer add onion and chiles. Stir-fry the onions until they start to brown around the edges, about 2 minutes.

Stir in the bok choy stems and stir-fry for 1 minute.

Add the beaten eggs and cook until it's nearly cooked through about 2 minutes, stirring often.

Stir in bok choy greens, basil and lime juice. And stir-fry for 30 seconds or so, until the greens are wilted. Serve immediately.

4. Skinny Eggie Vegetable Stir Fry

Ingredients:
1 lb of Cubed Butternut Squash
1 lb of Green Beans
3 Baby Bok Choys
1½ lb of Eggplants
3 Garlic Cloves
1 small Yellow Onion
½ teaspoon of low sodium salt
½ teaspoon of Black Pepper
1-2 Tablespoons of coconut oil
3 organic eggs

Instructions:

Peel, core, and cut the butternut squash into 1" cubes.

Snap the ends off the green beans and slice at an angle into 1.5" long pieces.

Chop the bok choy leaves from the stems. Slice the stems into 1" thick pieces. Cut the leaves in half.

Slice the eggplants into 1" thick discs, then quarter the disc into wedges. Slice in half if the eggplant is skinny.

Mince the garlic cloves and slice the onions.

Heat a wok and add the cooking oil.

Add the onions and cook until translucent. About 2 minutes.

Add the garlic and cook for another minute.

Add the squash, beans, low sodium salt, pepper

Add the eggplant and bok choy stalks and cook uncovered for another 7-10 minutes.

Add the bok choy leaves and cook for another few minutes, covered.

Beat the eggs and add them to the stir fry …keep stirring till they are cooked through

5. Rucola Salad

Ingredients:
4 teaspoons fresh lemon juice
4 teaspoons walnut oil
low sodium salt and freshly ground pepper
6 cups rucola leaves and tender stems (about 6 ounces)
Garlic powder to taste

Instructions:
Pour the lemon juice into a large bowl. Gradually whisk in the oil. Season with low sodium salt and pepper.

Add the greens, toss until evenly dressed and serve at once. This is delicious, and feel free to add tomatoes or grated carrot and onion slices.

Substitution: Any mild green, such as lamb's lettuce will do.

6. Tasty Spring Salad

Ingredients:
5 cups of any salad greens in season of your choice

Dressing:
125 mL (1/2 cup) olive oil
45 mL (3 tbsp) lemon juice
15 mL (1 tbsp) pure mustard powder
45 mL (3 tbsp) capers, minced (optional)
low sodium salt
pepper

Instructions:
Combine salad greens and any other raw vegetables of choice.

Combine oil, lemon juice and mustard. Mix well.

Add capers, low sodium salt and pepper to taste.

Pour dressing over salad, toss and serve.

7. Spinach and Dandelion Pomegranate Salad

Ingredients:
1 small bunch fresh spinach
12 dandelion leaves
1 cup pomegranate seeds
1/2 cup pecan halves

Instructions:
You may substitute appropriate fresh greens for the dandelion and sorrel leaves.

Wash and destem spinach. Pick and wash sorrel and dandelions.

Coarsely chop dandelion leaves, and tear spinach, then toss dandelion, sorrel and spinach together in a stainless steel bowl.

Put aside in refrigerator to drain and cool.

When drained, pour off excess water, and add pomegranate and pecans. Toss with dressing and serve.

8. Pure Delish Spinach Salad

Ingredients:
2 bunches fresh spinach
1 bunch scallions, chopped
juice of 1 lemon
1/4 tbsp olive oil
pepper to taste

optional: rice vinegar to taste

Instructions:
Wash spinach well. Drain and chop.

After a few minutes, squeeze excess water.

Add scallions, lemon juice, oil and pepper.

9. Sexy Salsa Salad

Ingredients:
1 bunch of cilantro
5-6 roma tomatoes
1 small yellow or red onion
1 small chili pepper
2 ripe avocados.
handful of rucola leaf

Instructions:
Chop cilantro, dice tomatoes, dice onion, finely dice chili pepper, dice avocado.

After dicing each ingredient add to large bowl. Add rucola to bowl.

When finished, toss.

10. Eastern Avo Salad

Ingredients:
2 to 3 lbs. of tomatoes
4 med. or lg. avocados (or 1lb chopped or ground nuts or seeds)
4 stalks celery
4 lg. red (or green) bell peppers
2 lbs. bok choy stalks and greens

Instructions:
Dice the tomatoes, celery and the bell peppers.

Quarter, peel and dice the avocados.

Cut up the bok choy.

Place all ingredients in a bowl and mix together.

11. Curry Coconut Salad

Ingredients:
6 large ripe tomatoes, peeled, seeded and chopped
1 small white onion, grated
1/4 tsp. coarsely ground pepper
1/2 cup coconut cream
2 Tbsp minced fresh parsley
1 tsp. curry powder

Instructions:
Combine tomatoes, onion and pepper; cover and chill for 3 hours.

Combine coconut cream, parsley and curry; cover and chill for 3 hours.

To serve, spoon tomato mixture into small bowls and top each with a spoonful of coconut cream mixture.

12. Jalapeno Salsa

Ingredients:
1 jalapeno pepper seeded and chopped fine
2 large ripe tomatoes, peeled and chopped
1 medium onion, minced
2 tbsp olive oil
juice of 1 lemon
1/2 tsp dried oregano
pepper to taste

Instructions:
Combine all ingredients and mix well. Refrigerate covered until ready to eat.

13. Beet Sprout Divine Salad

Ingredients:
1/2 pound Brussels sprouts, ends trimmed, outer leaves removed, and cut in half lengthwise
4 small red beets, tops trimmed to 1/2-inch, washed and cut in half lengthwise
4 tablespoons plus 1/3 cup extra virgin olive oil
1 tablespoon paleo Dijon mustard
Stevia to taste
Squeeze of lemon juice
Coarse low sodium salt
Grinding coarse black pepper
1 small red onion thinly sliced into rings

Instructions:
Preheat the oven to 350.

Pour 2 tablespoons olive oil in a baking dish. Toss the Brussels sprouts in the oil; sprinkle them with low sodium salt and pepper and roast them for 20 minutes.

Turn them once during the cooking. They are done when a small knife easily pierces them.

Pour 2 tablespoons of the olive oil on a sheet of aluminum foil and place

it on a baking sheet. Toss the beet halves in the olive oil. Sprinkle them with low sodium salt and pepper and, keeping them in a single layer, fold and seal the foil over them. Bake on the baking sheet until a knife easily pierces them.

When cool enough to handle, peel the beets and cut them into 1/4-inch slices.

Meanwhile combine the 1/3 cup olive oil, mustard, stevia, lemon juice and low sodium salt and pepper in a small bowl.

Toss the Ingredients, add the dressing and serve at room temperature.

14. Divine Carrot Salad

Ingredients:
3 tablespoons fresh lemon juice
1 tablespoon Olive oil
1 pressed garlic clove
1-1/2 pound carrots, peeled and rectangle and lightly steamed

Instructions:
Mix dressing ingredients in a small bowl. Add carrots; toss to mix.

Let stand at room temperature for one hour and then serve.

15. Cauliflower Couscous

Ingredients:
1 1/2 Lbs cauliflower florets
1/2 cup parsley (VERY finely chopped)
1/2 cup fresh mint (very FINELY chopped)
1/2 cup chopped red onion
One cucumber finely cubed
4.5 to 5 Tbls fresh lime juice (about 2 fruits)
2 Tbls olive oil
1 teas low sodium salt
1 teas black pepper

Instructions:
In a food processor (NOT A BLENDER) pulse cauliflower until it looks like rice. Set aside in serving bowl

In food processor- blend parsley, mint, onion, lime juice, olive oil, and low sodium salt and pepper into a smooth paste.

Pour over cauliflower and cucumber and blend well.

16. Mouthwatering Mushroom Salad

Ingredients:
2/3 cup olive oil
1/3 cup fresh lemon juice
One tablespoon red wine vinegar
1 tsp dried thyme
pepper and garlic powder to taste
1 pound fresh mushrooms, thinly sliced
1/4 cup minced parsley
Rucola leaves

Instructions:
Combine all ingredients except the mushrooms, parsley and greens, and mix well.

Add the mushrooms and toss with 2 forks. Cover and let stand at room temperature.

At serving time, drain and sprinkle with the parsley. Pile in a serving dish lined with greens.

17. Skinny Sweet Potato Salad

Ingredients:
4 small sweet potatoes
1 tablespoon olive oil extra virgin
1 teaspoon mustard powder
4 celery stalks, sliced 1/4-inch thick
1 small red bell pepper, cut into 1/4-inch dice
2 scallions, finely chopped
low sodium salt and pepper
1/2 cup coarsely chopped toasted pecans
Chopped fresh chives

Instructions:
Preheat oven to 400°F.

Wrap each sweet potato in foil and bake for 1 hour.

Unwrap; let cool. Peel; cut into 3/4-inch chunks.

In a large bowl, mix oil and mustard. Add sweet potatoes, celery, red pepper and scallions; toss gently.

Season to taste with low sodium salt and pepper.

Cover and refrigerate about 1 hour.

Fold in pecans and sprinkle with chives.

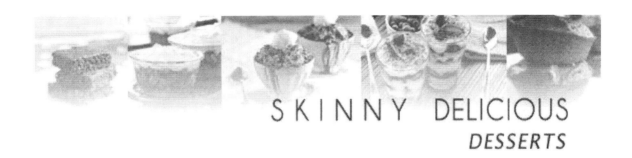

Paleo Epigenetic Desserts

1. Fabulous Brownie Treats

Ingredients:
1 1/2 cups walnuts
Pinch of low sodium salt
1 tsp vanilla
1/3 cup unsweetened cocoa powder
Stevia to taste

Instructions:

Add walnuts and low sodium salt to a blender or food processor. Mix until the walnuts are finely ground.

Add the vanilla, and cocoa powder etc to the blender. Mix well until everything is combined.

With the blender still running, add a couple drops of water at a time to make the mixture stick together.

Using a spatula, transfer the mixture into a bowl. Using your hands, form small round balls, rolling in your palm.

2. Rose Banana Delicious Brownies

Ingredients:
2 red beets, cooked
2 bananas
2 eggs
1/2 cup unsweetened cacao powder
1/3 cup almond flour
1 tsp baking powder
3 tablespoons crushes mixed nuts
Stevia to taste

Instructions:
Combine all ingredients in a food processor, and blend until smooth.

- Stir in the nut bits

Pour into a well-greased pan about 8x8 inches

Bake at 325 for about 40 minutes.

3. Pristine Pumpkin Divine

Ingredients:
2 cups blanched almond flour
½ cup flaxseed meal
2 teaspoons ground cinnamon (optional)
Stevia to taste
½ teaspoon low sodium salt
1 egg
1 cup pumpkin puree
1 tablespoon vanilla extract

Instructions:
Mix together the almond flour, flaxseed meal, cinnamon, and low sodium salt

In a separate bowl, whisk the egg, pumpkin and vanilla extract using a rubber spatula.

Gently mix dry and wet ingredients to form a batter being careful not to over mix or the batter will get oily and dense.

Spoon the batter onto a 9-inch pan lined with parchment paper or grease the pan

bake at 350°F until a toothpick inserted into the center comes out clean, approximately 25 minutes.

4. Secret Brownies

Ingredients:
1 c. raw almonds
1/2 c. raw cashews
4-5 Tbs. cocoa powder
1 Tbs. cashew butter
Stevia to taste

Instructions:
Combine all ingredients in the food processor.

Whir until somewhat smooth.

Press into 8×8" glass baking dish.

Chill until ready to serve.

5. Spectacular Spinach Brownies

Ingredients:
1 ¼ cups frozen chopped spinach
6 oz sugar free chocolate
½ cup extra virgin coconut oil
½ cup coconut oil
6 eggs
Stevia to taste
½ cup cocoa powder
1 Tspn vanilla pod
¼ tsp baking soda
½ tsp low sodium salt
½ tsp cream of tartar
pinch cinnamon

Instructions:

Preheat oven to 325F. Line a 9"x13" baking pan with wax paper or use a silicone baking pan.

Melt coconut oil and chocolate together over low heat on the stove top or medium power in the microwave. Add vanilla and stir to incorporate. Let cool.

Mix cocoa powder, baking soda, cream of tartar, low sodium salt and cinnamon.

Blend spinach, egg, together in a food processor or blender, until completely smooth (2-4 minutes).

Add coconut oil to food processor and process until full incorporated.

Add melted chocolate mixture and 3 or 4 drops stevia liquid to egg mixture slowly and processing/blending constantly.

Mix in dry ingredients and process/stir to fully incorporate.

Pour batter into prepared baking pan and spread out with a spatula.

Bake for 40 minutes. Cool completely in pan. Cut into squares. Enjoy!

6. Choco-coco Brownies

Ingredients:
6 Tablespoons of coconut oil
6 ounces of Sugar free Chocolate
4 Tablespoons of Packed Coconut Flour (20g)
¼ cup of Unsweetened Cocoa Powder (30g)
2 Eggs
½ teaspoon of Baking Soda
¼ teaspoon of low sodium salt
Extra coconut oil for pan greasing
Stevia to taste

Instructions:

Preheat the oven to 350F. Grease an 8x8 baking pan and line with parchment paper.

Ensure eggs are at room temperature. You may run them under warm water for about 10 seconds while shelled.

Gently melt the semisweet chocolate and oil in a double boiler. You may use the microwave at 50% heat at 30 second intervals with intermittent stirring.

Stir in unsweetened cocoa powder.

Sift together the superfine coconut flour, baking soda, stevia and low sodium salt.

Beat the eggs and add the dry ingredients. Beat until combined

Add the rest of the wet ingredients and beat until incorporated.

Pour the batter into the lined 8x8 pan.

Bake for 25-30 minutes at 350F until a toothpick inserted into the center of the batter comes out clean.

When done, remove from the oven and let cool in the pan for at least 15 minutes.

7. Coco – Walnut Brownie Bites

Ingredients:
2/3 cup raw walnut halves and pieces
1/3 cup unsweetened cocoa powder
1 tablespoon vanilla extract
1 to 2 tablespoons coconut milk
2/3 cups shredded unsweetened coconut

Instructions:

Pulse coconut in food processor for 30 seconds to a minute to form coconut crumbs. Remove from food processor and set aside.

Add unsweetened cocoa powder and walnuts to food processor, blend until walnuts become fine crumbs, but do not over process or you will get some kind of chocolate walnut butter.

Place in the food processor the cocoa walnut crumbs. Add vanilla. Process until mixture starts to combine.

Add coconut milk. You will know the consistency is right when the dough combines into a ball in the middle of the food processor.

If dough is too runny add a tablespoon or more cocoa powder to bring it back to a dough like state.

Transfer dough to a bowl and cover with plastic wrap. Refrigerate for at least 2 hours. Cold dough is much easier to work with. I left my dough in the fridge over night. You could put it in the freezer if you need to speed the process up.

Roll the dough balls in coconut crumbs, pressing the crumbs gently into the ball. Continue until all dough is gone.

8. Best Ever Banana Surprise Cake

Ingredients:
Bottom Fruit Layer:
2 tbsps coconut oil, melted
1 small banana, sliced, or ¼ cup blueberries for low carb version
2 tbsps walnut pieces * optional, can omit for nut free.
Stevia to taste
1 tsp ground cinnamon.

Top Cake Layer:
2 eggs, beaten.
Stevia to taste
¼ cup unsweetened coconut milk, or unsweetened almond milk.
1 tsp organic GF vanilla extract, or 1 tsp ground vanilla bean
½ tsp baking soda.
1 tsp apple cider vinegar.
1 small banana, mashed, or ¼ cup blueberries for lower carb version.
⅓ cup coconut flour

Instructions:
Preheat oven to 350 F, and lightly grease a 9 inch cake pan.

Place 2 tbsps coconut oil into cake pan, and put pan into preheating oven for a couple minutes to melt butter or oil. Once melted, make sure butter or oil is evenly distributed all over the bottom of the pan.

Sprinkle 2-4 drops stevia sweetener all over the melted oil.

Sprinkle 1 tsp cinnamon on top of sweetener layer.

Layer banana slices or blueberries on top of butter- sweetener layer, as seen in photo above. Add optional walnut pieces to fruit layer. Set aside.

In a large mixing bowl combine all the "top cake layer" ingredients except for the coconut flour. Mix thoroughly, then add the coconut flour and mix well, scraping sides of bowl, and braking up any coconut flour clumps.

Spoon cake batter on top of fruit layer in cake pan

Spread cake batter evenly across entire pan.

Bake for 25 minutes or until top of cake is browned and center is set.

Remove from oven and let cool completely.

Use a butter knife between cake and edge of pan and slide around to loosen cake from pan. Turn cake pan upside down onto a large plate or serving platter.

Slice and serve.

Should be stored in fridge, if serving later.

9. Choco Cookie Delight

Ingredients:
1/2 cup dark chocolate sugar free chips
1/2 cup coconut milk (thick fat from top of can)
2 eggs
1 cup almond flour
pinch of low sodium salt
1/2 teaspoon vanilla extract
1/4 teaspoon baking powder

Vanilla glaze:
1/2 cup coconut butter, liquid
Stevia to taste
1 /2 teaspoon vanilla extract

Chocolate Glaze:
1/2 cup chocolate chips
Stevia powder for decoration

Instructions:
Place a small sauce pan over low heat and melt your chocolate and coconut milk together (only keep the heat on long enough to melt them together)

While melting, place your 2 eggs in a stand mixer with the whisk, or use a hand mixer with the whisk and beat your eggs until they are fluffy, about 1 minute

Add your coconut milk and chocolate to your eggs and mix well

Stir in your almond flour, low sodium salt, vanilla extract and baking powder

Mix well ensuring everything is combined

Pipe your batter into the cookie wells ensuring you fill higher than the halfway point

Remove from the cookie maker, gently insert the sticks and place everything in the freezer for 30-45 minutes

Vanilla Glaze:

Combine your coconut butter, stevia, and vanilla extract in a small glass to make it easy to dip

You can keep this glass in hot water to keep the glaze more liquidy to make the dipping easier

Chocolate Glaze:

Melt your chocolate chips over a double boiler and keep the heat low and them liquid – then spread over cooled cookies!

10. Choco Triple Delight

Ingredients:
Cake:
1 cup almond flour (or 3 oz ground raw pumpkin seeds for nut-free version)
3 tbsp Raw Cacao Powder
1 tbsp coconut flour
1 tsp baking powder
1/2 tsp baking soda
1/8th tsp Stevia
3 tbsp melted Raw Cacao Butter or coconut oil)
Pinch of low sodium salt
1 large pastured egg
2 tbsp coconut milk (or dairy of choice)
1 tsp pure vanilla extract
2 oz 80% cocoa bar, chopped
Top with 2 tbsp chopped nut of choice,
Optional: 1/8th tsp low sodium salt sprinkled on top of cake before baking

Chocolate Drizzle:
2 tbsp coconut cream concentrate, warmed
3 tbsp water (or coconut milk)
3 tbsp Cacao powder
1/2 tbsp pure vanilla extract
Stevia to taste

Instructions:
Preheat oven to 350 degrees F.

Oil the sides and bottom of 8 inch cake pan.

Line the bottom of the pan with parchment paper and set aside.

In a medium bowl, add dry ingredients. Use a sifter to insure that all ingredients are blended well and that there are no lumps.

Add remaining ingredients (except nuts and optional salt) to dry ingredients and mix. Taste for sweetness and adjust if necessary.

Press (or spread with angled spatula) into a 8 inch cake pan. Sprinkle with nuts. Bake for 11-14 minutes.

DO NOT OVER BAKE! Remove from oven and serve warm or allow to cool and top with Chocolate Drizzle.

Chocolate Drizzle:

In a small bowl, blend coconut cream concentrate and water until smooth.

Add cacao powder, vanilla and stevia. Whisk until creamy.

Taste for sweetness and adjust if necessary. Drizzle over the cake.

11. Peach and Almond Cake

Ingredients:
2 whole peaches
300g almond meal
6 eggs
Stevia to taste
1 tsp baking soda

Instructions:
Cover the peaches in water in a saucepan and boil for about 2 hours.

Preheat the oven to 180 degrees Celsius and line the bottom of a 24cm pan with baking paper.

Lightly beat the eggs.

Blend the eggs and peaches (quarter them first) thoroughly in a food processor.

Add the rest of the ingredients to the food processor, again blending thoroughly.

Pour mixture into the lined tin and bake for roughly an hour.

12. Apple Cinnamon Walnut Bonanza

Ingredients:
For the cake:
1 cup almond flour
2 tablespoons coconut flour
Stevia to taste
1 tablespoon cinnamon
1 teaspoon baking soda
1/4 teaspoon low sodium salt
1 tablespoon coconut butter, plus more for greasing the pan
2 eggs
1/2 cup cream from a can of refrigerated coconut milk
1 teaspoon vanilla
1 cup grated apple (about 1 large apple)

For the topping:
1 1/2 cups walnuts (or pecans, if you prefer)
1/2 cup almond flour
4 tablespoons melted coconut butter
Stevia to taste
1 tablespoon cinnamon
pinch low sodium salt

Instructions:
Preheat your oven to 350° and grease a 8 x 8 baking dish.

<u>Make the topping:</u> pulse the walnuts in a food processor 10-12 times or until they are course crumbs. Add the remaining ingredients and pulse 2-3 more times until combined. Set aside.

Wipe out and dry the bowl of your food processor and add your dry **cake** ingredients. (almond flour through low sodium salt) Pulse a few times to mix.

Cut the tablespoon of butter into smaller chunks and add it to the dry ingredients. Pulse 8-10 times or until it's cut in to the dry ingredients, similar to if you were making a pie crust.

In a small bowl, mix your wet cake ingredients (eggs through vanilla) and whisk until well combined. Stir in grated apple.

Add to the food processor and mix until combined. Scrape down the sides once or twice to make sure it's well mixed.

Pour into the prepared baking dish and sprinkle the topping over, as evenly as you can.

Bake for 30-35 minutes, or until a toothpick inserted into the center comes out clean.

Allow to cool, and enjoy!

13. Chestnut- Cacao Cake

Ingredients:
100g (1 cup + 1 heaping tablespoon) chestnut flour
50g (1/2 cup) ground almonds (almond flour)
3 eggs, separate
1/2 teaspoon cream of tartar
35g (1/2 cup) raw cacao powder
Stevia to taste
3/4 cup coconut milk
1/2 teaspoon baking soda
Crushed chesnuts

Instructions:
Preheat oven to 180C fan (350F).

Grease a pie/tart pan.

In a clean mixing bowl, beat the egg whites and cream of tartar until stiff peaks form. Set aside.

In another mixing bowl, cream the egg yolks, chestnut flour, ground almonds, stevia, raw cacao, baking soda and coconut milk.

Fold in the egg whites and blend until the white is no longer showing.

Pour into the pie/tart mold.

Sprinkle with crushed chestnuts, if desired.

Bake for 35-40 minutes on the middle rack.

14. Extra Dark Choco Delight

Ingredients:
1 egg
½ very ripe avocado
¼ cup full fat canned coconut milk
2 tbsp cacao powder
1 tbsp carob powder
pinch low sodium salt
pinch cinnamon
1 scoop vanilla flavored hemp protein powder
10g raw hazelnuts
2 tbsp unsweetened shredded coconut
Stevia to taste

Instructions:
Add the egg, avocado and coconut milk to a small food processor and process until very smooth and process until very smooth and creamy.

Add cacao powder, carob powder, low sodium salt, cinnamon and protein powder and process again until well combined and creamy.

Add hazelnuts and shredded coconut and give a few extra spins until the hazelnuts are reduced to tiny little pieces.

Serve immediately or refrigerate until ready to serve.

Garnish with a little dollop of coconut cream and cacao nibs or shredded coconut and crushed hazelnuts.

This will keep in the refrigerator for a few days in an airtight container.

15. Nut Butter Truffles

Ingredients:
5 tablespoons sunflower seed butter
1 tablespoon coconut oil
2 teaspoons vanilla extract
¾ cup almond flour
1 tablespoon flaxseed meal
pinch of low sodium salt
¼ cup sugar free dark chocolate chips
1 tablespoon cacao butter
chopped almonds (optional)
stevia to taste

Instructions:

Add sunflower seed butter, coconut oil, vanilla, almond flour, flaxseed meal and low sodium salt to a large bowl. Please note that you may find a thin layer of oil in the sunflower seed butter jar that separates from the butter and rises to the top. Be sure to mix oil and butter together before scooping into bowl.

Using your hands mix until all ingredients are incorporated (I like using gloves when mixing so the oils from my skin do not get into the mixture)

Roll the dough into 1-inch balls and place them on a sheet of parchment paper and refrigerate for 30 minutes (using 2 teaspoons for each truffle will yield about 14 truffles)

Melt the chocolate chips in a double boiler along with the cacao butter

Dip each truffle in the melted chocolate, one at the time, and place them back on the pan with parchment paper

Top with chopped almonds and refrigerate until the chocolate is firm

16. Fetching Fudge

Ingredients:
1 cup coconut butter
1/4 cup coconut oil
1/4 cup cocoa
1/4 cup cocoa powder + 1 Tbsp
Stevia to taste
1 tsp vanilla

Instructions:

In the pot, gently melt the cocoa butter on low (number 2)

When it is half melted add the butter, the coconut oil and the coconut spread and gently mix with the whisk as it melts

Add vanilla, and stevia and whisk in well

Add the cocoa powder and whisk in well

Be sure to take the pot off the heat when the fat is melted and keep whisking until it is smooth and all the lumps are out — you don't want to overheat this

Pour into the 8 x 8 pan that is lined with parchment paper

Refrigerate for 1 – 2 hours

When solid, pull the parchment paper out of the pan, put the block of fudge on a flat surface and cut into small squares

Enjoy! This will melt rather quickly — but it won't last long!

17. Choco – Almond Delights

Ingredients:
1 c. toasted hazelnuts
1 c. raw almonds
2/3 c. raw almond butter
5 Tbs. raw cacao powder (or unsweetened cocoa powder)
1/2 tsp. vanilla extract
1/4 c. unsweetened, shredded coconut
Stevia to taste

Instructions:
Combine all the ingredients, except for the coconut, in the food processor. Whir until smooth. This will take a few minutes and may require scraping down the sides of the bowl one or more times.

Line a mini muffin tin with plastic wrap. Spoon dollops of the sweet mixture into the lined tin cups and form into "mounds." Freeze until well formed. Remove mounds from plastic and tin and flip for presentation. Sprinkle with shredded coconut.

18. Chococups

Ingredients:
4 eggs
Stevia to taste
1/3 cup coconut flour
1/4 cup cacao powder
1/2 teaspoon baking soda
1/4 cup coconut oil (melted in microwave)
1/4 cup cacao butter (melted in microwave)

For topping:
1 can coconut cream (chilled in fridge overnight)
Cacao nibs to decorate.

Instructions:
Heat oven to 170 degrees Celsius (338F)

Grease 10 muffin pans with coconut oil.

Beat eggs with electric beaters.

Add coconut flour, baking soda and cacao powder.

Beat well and add stevia

Add melted coconut oil, cacao butter and mix.

Spoon mixture into 10 greased muffin pans.

Bake for 12-15 minutes until risen and top springs back.

Cool in pans.

Beat the solid coconut cream with electric beaters until creamy. Add honey to taste if you wish.

Pipe coconut cream onto top of cakes.

19. Choco Coco Cookies

Ingredients:
Stevia powder – 1 teaspoon – or to taste
1 cup coconut flour
½ cup coconut oil
½ cup coconut milk, (from the can)
2 Teaspoons vanilla extract
¼ Teaspoon low sodium salt
2½ cups finely shredded coconut
1 cup big flake coconut
⅔ cup dark sugar free chocolate chunks or chocolate chips (I used 80% dark chocolate)
Optional: ½ cup almond or cashew butter

Instructions:

In a large saucepan, combine the, coconut oil, and coconut milk. Bring the mixture to a boil, and boil for 2-3 minutes.

Remove from the heat and add the vanilla, low sodium salt, and coconut flour and coconut. Stir to combine. If you're using the almond or cashew butter, mix it in thoroughly. Finally, add the chocolate chunks and combine, stirring as little as possible to keep the chunks intact.

Portion the cookie on a parchment lined baking sheet and let cool. This version of no-bakes takes a full 3-4 hours to fully set up, but you don't have to wait that long because they're really good warm and gooey.

20. Apple Spice Spectacular

Ingredients:
1 cup unsweetened almond butter
Stevia to taste
1 egg
1 tsp baking soda
1/2 tsp low sodium salt
half an apple, diced 1 tsp cinnamon
1/4 tsp ground cloves
1/8 tsp nutmeg
1 tsp fresh ginger, grated on a microplane

Instructions:
Pre-heat oven to 350 degress F.

In a large bowl, combine almond butter, stevia, egg, baking soda, and low sodium salt until well incorporated. Add apple, spices, and ginger and stir to combine.

Spoon batter onto a baking sheet (you may have to spread the batter a little to get it into a round shape) about 1-2 inches apart from each other--they'll spread a bit.

Bake about 10 minutes, or until slightly set.

Remove cookies and allow to cool on pan for about 5-10 minutes. Then finish cooling on a cooling rack.

21. Absolute Almond Bites

Ingredients:
1 1/2 cups almond flour
1/4 teaspoon low sodium salt
1/4 teaspoon baking soda (gluten-free, if necessary)
1/8 teaspoon cinnamon
2 tablespoons melted coconut oil
Stevia to taste
1 1/4 teaspoon vanilla extract
1/4 teaspoon almond extract or almond flavoring
12 to 15 whole almonds; sprouted or soaked and dehydrated

Instructions:

Preheat oven to 325°F. Line a baking sheet with parchment paper.

In a medium bowl combine almond flour, low sodium salt, baking soda, and cinnamon. Mix well, breaking up any lumps.

In a small bowl, place coconut oil, vanilla, almond extract or flavoring. Whisk until well combined.

Add wet ingredients to dry ingredients and stir until combined…add stevia

Roll level-tablespoon-sized (using a measuring spoon) portions of dough into balls and place on baking sheet. Flatten slightly with the heel of your hand and press one almond into the center of each cookie.

Bake 15 to 17 minutes or until light golden brown. Allow to cool on baking sheet for a few minutes before transferring to cooling rack.

Store in an airtight container. Can be frozen.

22. Eastern Spice Delights

Ingredients:
1 3/4 cups + 4 tbsp almond meal
1/8 tsp low sodium salt
3/4 tsp ground ginger
3/4 tsp cinnamon
1/4 tsp ground cloves
1/4 tsp cardamom
1/8 tsp nutmeg
1/2 cup coconut oil (in solid form)
Stevia to taste
1 tsp vanilla extract

Instructions:
Preheat oven to 350F.

Combine all the dry ingredients in a large bowl. In a small bowl, mix together the oil, maple syrup, and vanilla until completely blended. Pour the wet ingredients over the dry ingredients and mix well.

Drop the cookie dough on a cookie sheet. It will spread a bit as it cooks (and thus flatten), but not an awful lot.

Bake for 10-12 minutes. These cookies will not look golden when they're done. Makes two dozens.

23. Berry Ice Cream and Almond Delight

Ingredients:
For the Ice Cream:
1 can full fat coconut milk
Stevia to taste
2 tbsp vanilla
1 cup fresh strawberries, cut into fourths

For the crisp:
1/3 cup almond flour
3 tbsp sunflower seed butter (or almond butter)
1/2 tsp vanilla
1 tbsp honey
low sodium salt to taste

Instructions:
For the ice cream:

Combine coconut milk and vanilla together in a small saucepan over medium heat and stir until ingredients are well combined (just a few minutes).

Transfer milk mixture to a small bowl and place in the freezer for two hours.

Next, add strawberries to a small saucepan and bring to a low boil.

Turn heat to medium-low and allow to cook until they start breaking down into a sauce-like mixture, leaving small chunks.

Place strawberries in refrigerator while the ice cream hardens.

For the crisp:

Combine all ingredients and mix until you get a "crumble' consistency.

Place crisp in refrigerator until ready to use.

After two hours, place milk mixture into your ice cream maker along with the strawberries and use as directed.

When ice cream is ready, scoop and serve with crisp sprinkled on top.

24. Creamy Caramely Ice Cream

Ingredients:
Delicious Instant Caramel Topping:
2 heaped tablespoons of hulled tahini
Stevia to taste
2 tablespoons of coconut milk
1/2 teaspoon of vanilla

Delicious Instant Ice Cream:
4 frozen bananas, chopped
4 tablespoons coconut milk
1 teaspoon of vanilla

Instructions:
Spoon the tahini and stevia into a cup and stir with a fork to combine. Mix in the coconut milk and vanilla. Refrain from eating it while you make your ice cream.

Place the ingredients into food processor or blender, blend until the mixture is an ice cream consistency.

Spoon the ice cream into bowls, drizzle generously with the caramel topping, sprinkle with low sodium salt if you desire. Enjoy!

25. Cheeky Cherry Ice

Ingredients:
14oz. cans 365 Coconut Milk (Full Fat)
Stevia to taste
1 ½ tsp. vanilla extract
2 cups fresh cherries, pitted and diced

Instructions:

In a large bowl, combine coconut milk, stevia and vanilla and stir well.

Chill for 1-2 hours.

Transfer to ice-cream maker and process according to manufacturer directions.

Add diced cherries to the mixture during the last 5-10 minutes of processing.

26. Choco - Coconut Berry Ice

Ingredients:
Follow recipe of berry ice cream and almond delight for the ice cream only
4 ounces sugar free dark chocolate - 75% cacao content
¼ cup coconut milk
2 cups fresh berries (I used raspberries)
Stevia to taste

Instructions:
Make the Homemade Coconut Ice Cream,

While the ice cream is freezing in the machine, break the chocolate into pieces and place in a small saucepan.

Add the coconut milk and melt the two together, stirring over low heat.

When the chocolate mixture is completely smooth, pour the chocolate over the ice cream and stir to create 'ripples'. If your ice cream if thoroughly frozen, soften in the fridge for 20 minutes before stirring in the chocolate.

Serve immediately with the fresh berries, or freeze for an additional 3-4 hours for a firmer texture.

27. Creamy Berrie Pie

Ingredients:
Crust:
3 cups almonds
½ Teaspoon cinnamon
½ cup honey
2 Tablespoons coconut oil
1 Tablespoon lemon zest
1 Teaspoon almond extract
pinch of low sodium salt

Filling:
2 Teaspoons plant-based gelatin, dissolved in 2 Tablespoons hot water
⅓ cup freshly squeezed lemon juice
Stevia to taste
1 can coconut milk, chilled
4 cups blueberries for serving

Instructions:
Place the almonds and cinnamon in a food processor and pulse until your desired texture is reached. I like to leave some bigger pieces for texture. Add the rest of the crust ingredients and pulse until a sticky dough forms. Pat the crust into a pie plate, (use water to keep your hands from sticking to the crust).

For the filling, mix the gelatin and water together. Stir to dissolve and immediately add the lemon juice. If the gelatin gets clumpy, place the mixture over hot water until it melts again. Pour the coconut milk into an electric mixer, add the stevia and whip on high until peaks form, about 15 minutes. Add the gelatin mixture to the whipped cream. Pour the filling into the crust. The filling will seem thin, but don't worry it will set up in the refrigerator.

Chill for at least 4 hours until set, and serve with lots of berries!

28. Peachy Creamy Peaches

Ingredients:
3 medium ripe peaches, cut in half with pit removed
1 tsp vanilla
1 can coconut milk, refrigerated
1/4 cup chopped walnuts
Cinnamon and stevia (to taste)

Instructions:
Place peaches on the grill with the cut side down first. Grill on medium-low heat until soft, about 3-5 minutes on each side.

Scoop cream off the top of the can of chilled coconut milk. Whip together coconut cream and vanilla with handheld mixer. Drizzle over each peach. Top with cinnamon and chopped walnuts to garnish.

29. Spiced Apple Bake

Ingredients:
2 apples of your choice
1/4 cup walnuts
1/4 tablespoon nutmeg
1/4 tablespoon cinnamon
1/4 tablespoon ground cloves

Instructions:
Preheat oven to 350 degrees Fahrenheit.

Slice the very top and very bottom off of each apple. (The top allows for more room to stuff with goodies, the bottom allows the apples to soak up all the nice sauce).

Core both apples to the bottom, but not all the way through.

Mix spices, walnuts, and raisins in a small bowl.

Pour half of the spice mixture into each apple.

Place on baking sheet and bake 20-25 minutes, or until apples are soft. I like to pour any remaining sauce mixture into the bottom of the pan so the apples can soak up the flavors.

30. Sexy Dessert Pan

Ingredients:

Crust:
1 1/2 cups pecans
3/4 cup dates
4 tbsp coconut oil

Second Layer:
2/3 cup cashew butter
1/3 cup palm shortening
2 tsp apple cider vinegar
1/2 tsp lemon juice
Pinch low sodium salt

Third Layer:
1 cup coconut flour
1 cup coconut milk
Stevia to taste
1 tsp vanilla extract

Fourth Layer:
1/2 cup coconut milk
1/2 cup coconut butter
1/2 cup cacao powder
2 tbsp honey

Fifth Layer:
1/2 cup coconut butter
1/4 cup coconut milk
Stevia to taste

Sixth Layer:
Grated dark sugar free chocolate, at least 80% cacao

Instructions:

To make the crust, roughly chop the pecans then pit and chop the dates. Load both into a food processor and pulse until ground but still crumbly. Transfer to a bowl and work in the coconut oil, then press the sticky mixture into a single smooth layer at the bottom of a square 8x8 cake pan.

Transfer to the refrigerator to chill while you begin the second layer. To make the second layer, combine its ingredients very well in a medium mixing bowl. Spoon over the chilled crust, smoothing as much as possible with the back of a spoon. Place the pan back in the fridge.

To make the third layer, mix its ingredients together in a mixing bowl and then spoon over the chilled, hardened second layer. Smooth as much as possible, then chill.

Add the fourth layer by combining its ingredients and then layering it into the pan in the same way as the previous layers.

For the fifth layer, mix the coconut shortening, coconut milk and stevia with a hand mixer until very smooth and spoon over the chilled fourth layer.

Before placing the pan back into the refrigerator after adding the fifth layer, grate very dark chocolate over the top to the depth of your preference. Chill the pan for an additional half hour or more, then slice with a sharp knife and serve.

31. Pretty Pumpkin Delights

Ingredients:
For Crust:
1 cup hazelnuts (preferably soaked and dehydrated for better digestion)
1/2 cup raw pumpkin seeds (preferably soaked and dehydrated for better digestion)
1 TBS coconut oil
2 pinches of low sodium salt
Stevia to taste

For Filling:
1 cup cooked pumpkin puree
1/2 cup coconut
2 TBS coconut oil
Stevia to taste
1/2 tsp vanilla extract
1/4 tsp cinnamon powder
1/4 tsp ginger powder
1/8 tsp allspice
1/8 tsp clove powder

For Chocolate Drizzle:
2 TBS coconut butter
2 TBS coconut oil
2 TBS raw cacao (or unsweetened cocoa)
Stevia to taste
a pinch or 2 of low sodium salt

Instructions:
To Make the crust: Line mini muffin tins with unbleached mini paper liners. Process all crust ingredients in a food processor until well combined and resembles a coarse flour. Spoon 1 and 1/2 tsp of mixture into each of the 24 mini cups. Use your thumb to press down mixture firmly to create a solid bottom layer for these cute little yummies. Place in freezer to harden.

To make filling: Melt coconut butter and coconut oil in a double boiler. Remove from heat and add rest of filling ingredients. Go ahead and mix it up real good here until creamy smooth. Remove crusts from freezer and spoon about 3/4 TBS of filling over your prepared crusts. Return to freezer to harden, at least 2 hours.

To make chocolate drizzle: Once mini bites have hardened, gently melt coconut butter and coconut oil in a double boiler. Remove from heat and add rest of drizzle ingredients. Allow to cool slightly to thicken. Pour into small plastic bag, cut a TINY hole in the corner, and drizzle over treats in any fashion that you want.

Now it's time to enjoy these amazing delights. Store leftovers in freezer as they are best cold. (That is, if there are any leftovers. Ours got dusted off in one day.)

32. Macadamia Pineapple Bonanza

Ingredients:

Crust:
½ cup almond flour
4 tablespoons raw cacao powder
⅓ cup macadamia nuts
½ teaspoon vanilla extract
Stevia to taste
1½ teaspoons coconut oil, melted

Filling:
2 eggs
1 cup fresh pineapple, chopped
1⅓ cup shredded coconut, unsweetened
1 tablespoon fresh lime juice
1 tablespoon vanilla extract
Stevia to taste
½ cup almond flour
pinch of low sodium salt

Instructions:

Crust:

In a large bowl, mix the almond flour and cacao powder.

Chop the macadamia nuts in a food processor and add it to the bowl.

Add vanilla extract and coconut oil to the dry mixture and using your hands, mix to combine ingredients.

Spread the mixture evenly on the bottom of an 8x8-inch pan lined with parchment paper. Be sure to use one large piece of paper covering the entire pan that overlaps on all four sides.

Filing:

In a large bowl beat the 2 eggs

Mix in the pineapple, 1 cup of shredded coconut (reserve the remaining ⅓ cup for the top), lime juice, vanilla and stevia.

Gently mix in the almond flour and low sodium salt with rubber spatula.

Pour mixture over the crust and sprinkle top with remaining shredded coconut.

Bake at 350°F for approximately 20 minutes or until the top starts to brown and the pineapple/coconut layer is firm.

Set pan on a wire rack and allow it to cool before cutting into squares. Store in the refrigerator.

33. Lemony Lemon Delights

Ingredients:
Crust:
1 cup almond flour
1/4 cup almond butter
Stevia to taste
1 tbsp coconut butter
1 tsp vanilla
1/2 tsp baking powder
1/4 tsp low sodium salt

Filling:
3 eggs
Stevia to taste
1/4 cup lemon juice
2 1/2 tbsp coconut flour
1 tbsp lemon zest, finely grated
Pinch of low sodium salt

Instructions:
Preheat oven to 350.

Coat 9×9 baking dish with coconut oil or butter.

Combine all crust ingredients in food processor until a "crumble" forms.

Press crust evenly into the bottom of pan.

Using a fork, prick a few holes into crust.

Bake for 10 minutes.

While crust is baking, combine all filling ingredients in a food processor until well incorporated.

When done, remove crust from oven and pour filling evenly over top.

Continue to bake for 15-20 minutes, or until filling is set, but still has a little jiggle.

Cool completely on wire rack. (You can also chill in the fridge if desired, to further set the filling).

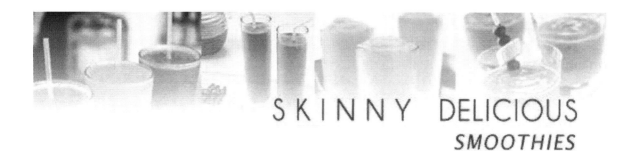

SKINNY DELICIOUS SMOOTHIES

Paleo Epigenetic Smoothies

1. Gorgeous Berry Smoothie

Ingredients:
½ cup frozen blueberries or 1 cup fresh blueberries
15 oz coconut milk
Stevia to taste
1 scoop of hemp protein
¼ teaspoon cinnamon (optional)

Instructions:
Place all ingredients into a blender.

Blend until mixed thoroughly.

Serve right away.

2. Tempting Coconut Berry Smoothie

Ingredients:
½ Cup Frozen Blackberries
½ Frozen Banana
1 Teaspoon Chia Seeds
¼ Inch Piece of Fresh Ginger
½ Cup Almond
Coconut Milk
1 scoop of HEMP protein
2 Tablespoons Toasted Coconut

Instructions:
Combine all the ingredients in a blender and process until smooth.

3. Volumptious Vanilla Hot Drink

Ingredients:
3 cups unsweetened almond milk (or 1 1/2 cup full fat coconut milk + 1 1/2 cups water)
Stevia to taste
1 scoop of hemp protein
1/2 Tbsp. ground cinnamon (or more to taste)
1/2 Tbsp. vanilla extract

Instructions:
Place the almond milk into a pitcher. Place ground cinnamon, hemp, anilla extract in a small saucepan over medium high heat. Heat until the pure liquid stevia is just melted and then pour the pure liquid stevia mixture into the pitcher.

Stir until the pure liquid stevia is well combined with the almond milk. Place the pitcher in the fridge and allow to chill for at least two hours. Stir well before serving.

4. Almond Butter Smoothies

Ingredients:
1 scoop of hemp protein
1 Tablespoon natural almond butter
1 cup of hemp milk
1 banana, preferably frozen for a creamier shake
few ice cubes

Instructions:
Blend all ingredients together and enjoy!

5. Choco Walnut Delight

Ingredients:
1 scoop Hemp Protein
30g dark sugar free chocolate broken up.
50g walnuts chopped/crushed (depending on desired texture)
250ml hemp milk or nut milk alternative
Handfull of ice cubes, the more you use the thicker it will be.

Instructions:
Blend everything together in a strong blender until thoroughly processed, and enjoy!

Makes 2, and can be stored in the fridge overnight.

6. Raspberry Hemp Smoothie

Ingredients:
1 cup hemp milk or milk alternative
1/2 cup raspberries (fresh or frozen)
2 tablespoons hemp protein powder
Stevia to taste
3 to 4 ice cubes

Instructions:
Add ingredients to a blender and blend until smooth.

7. Choco Banana Smoothie

Ingredients:
1 cup milk or milk alternative
2 peeled frozen bananas
4 ice cubes
2 tablespoons hulled hemp seed
2 tablespoons hemp protein powder
1 tablespoons organic cocoa powder
5-7 drops liquid stevia to sweeten
1/4 teaspoon cinnamon
1/4 teaspoon vanilla

Instructions:
Put all ingredients into blender. Blend until smooth.

8. Blueberry Almond Smoothie

Ingredients:
1 c almond milk
1 c frozen unsweetened blueberries
1 Tbsp cold-pressed organic flaxseed oil
2 tblsp hemp protein powder

Instructions:
Combine milk and blueberries in blender, and blend for 1 minute.

Transfer to glass, and stir in flaxseed oil.

9. Hazelnut Butter and Banana Smoothie

Ingredients:
½ c nut milk
½ c hemp milk
2 Tbsp creamy natural unsalted hazelnut butter
¼ very ripe banana
stevia drops to taste
4 ice cubes
2 tblsp hemp protein powder

Instructions:
Combine ingredients in a blender. Process until smooth.

Pour into a tall glass and serve.

10. Vanilla Blueberry Smoothie

Ingredients:
2 cups hemp milk
1 c fresh blueberries
Handful of ice OR 1 cup frozen blueberries
1 Tbsp flaxseed oil
2 tblsp hemp protein powder

Instructions:
Combine milk, and fresh blueberries plus ice (or frozen blueberries) in a blender.

Blend for 1 minute, transfer to a glass, and stir in flaxseed oil.

11. Chocolate Raspberry Smoothie

Ingredients:
1 cup almond milk
¼ c chocolate chips-sugar free
1 c fresh raspberries
2 tsp hemp protein powder
Handful of ice OR 1 cup frozen raspberries

Instructions:
COMBINE ingredients in a blender.

Blend for 1 minute, transfer to a glass, and eat with a spoon.

12. Peach Smoothie

Ingredients:
1 cup hemp milk
1 c frozen unsweetened peaches
2 tsp cold-pressed organic flaxseed oil (MUFA)
2 tsp hemp protein powder

Instructions:
PLACE milk and frozen, unsweetened peaches in blender and blend for 1 minute.

Transfer to glass, and stir in flaxseed oil.

13. Zesty Citrus Smoothie

Ingredients:
1 cup almond milk
half cup lemon juice
1 med orange peeled, cleaned, and sliced into sections
Handful of ice
1 Tbsp flaxseed oil
2 tsp hemp protein powder

Instructions:
COMBINE milk, lemon juice, orange, and ice in a blender.

Blend for 1 minute, transfer to a glass, and stir in flaxseed oil.

14. Apple Smoothie

Ingredients:
½ cup hemp milk
1 cup hemp milk
1 tsp apple pie spice
1 med apple peeled and chopped
2 Tbsp cashew butter
Handful of ice
2 tblsp hemp protein powder

Instructions:
COMBINE ingredients in a blender.

Blend for 1 minute, transfer to a glass, and eat with a spoon.

15. Pineapple Smoothie

Ingredients:
1 cup almond milk
4 oz fresh pineapple
Handful of ice
2 tblsp hemp protein powder
1 Tbsp cold-pressed organic flaxseed oil

Instructions:
PLACE milk, canned pineapple in blender, add of ice, and whip for 1 minute.

Transfer to glass and stir in flaxseed oil.

16. Strawberry Smoothie

Ingredients:
1 cup almond milk
1 c frozen, unsweetened strawberries
2 tblsp hemp protein powder
2 tsp cold-pressed organic flaxseed oil

Instructions:
COMBINE milk and strawberries in blender.

Blend, transfer to glass, and stir in flaxseed oil.

17. Pineapple Coconut Deluxe Smoothie

Ingredients:
1 C pineapple chunks
1 C coconut milk
1/2 C pineapple juice
1 ripe banana
1/2 – 3/4 C ice cubes
Pure liquid stevia to taste
1 tablespoon hemp protein powder

Instructions:
In a blender, combine the pineapple chunks, coconut milk, banana, ice and pure liquid stevia.

Puree until smooth.

Pour into 2 large glasses.

Garnish with a pineapple wedge if desired.

18. Divine Vanilla Smoothie

Ingredients:
1 cup coconut or almond milk
¼ cup almond butter
1 tsp vanilla paste, (or vanilla extract)
2 cups ice
Vanilla liquid, seeds or powder, to taste
Vanilla or plain hemp Protein Powder – 1 tablespoon

Instructions:
Add all ingredients except ice to blender. Puree well.

Add ice and blend until ice is all crushed and smoothie is well blended and smooth.

Pour into two glasses and serve immediately.

NOTES
Add more or less ice to make the smoothie thinner or thicker consistency.
Great for a post workout smoothie!

19. Coco Orange Delish Smoothie

Ingredients:
1/2 cup fresh squeezed orange juice (I used 1 1/2 oranges)
1 tablespoon hemp protein powder
1/2 cup full fat coconut milk from the can (not the box!)
1 teaspoon vanilla
1/2 -1 cup crushed ice

Instructions:
Add all ingredients to a blender.

Blend until smooth and add ice as needed to get the consistency you like.

20. Baby Kale Pineapple Smoothie

Ingredients:
1 cup almond milk
1/2 cup frozen pineapple
1 cup Kale
1 tablespoon hemp protein powder

Instructions:
Place the almond milk, pineapple, and greens in the blender and blend until smooth.

21. Sumptuous Strawberry Coconut Smoothie

Ingredients:
1 cup coconut milk
1 frozen banana, sliced
2 cups frozen strawberries
1 teaspoon vanilla extract
1 tablespoon hemp protein powder

Instructions:
Add all ingredients to blender and blend until smooth.

22. Blueberry Bonanza Smoothies

Ingredients:
1/4 cup canned coconut or almond milk
1/2 cup water
1 medium banana, sliced
1 cup frozen blueberries
1 tablespoon raw almonds

Instructions:
Add coconut milk, water, banana, blueberries and almonds to blender container.

Cover and blend until smooth. Pour into 2 glasses.

23. Divine Peach Coconut Smoothie

Ingredients:
1 cup full fat coconut milk, chilled
1 cup ice
2 large fresh peaches, peeled and cut into chunks
Fresh lemon zest, to taste
1 tablespoon hemp protein powder

Instructions:

Add coconut milk, ice and peaches blender. Using a zester, add a few gratings of fresh lemon zest.

Blend on high speed until smooth.

24. Tantalizing Key Lime Pie Smoothie

Ingredients:
1 cup coconut milk
1 cup ice
1/2 avocado
zest and juice of 2 limes
Pure liquid stevia to taste
1 tablespoon hemp protein powder

Instructions:
Add all ingredients to Vitamix or blender and blend until smooth.

25. High Protein and Nutritional Delish Smoothie

Ingredients:
1 cup almond milk
1/2 Avocado
4 Strawberries
1/2 Bananas (Very ripe)
1/2 cup Raw Kale or spinach
1/4 cup Carrot Juice) water can be used
1 cup Coconut Yogurt..or almond milk)
1 tablespoon hemp protein powder

Instructions:
Add everything to your blender, and blend to your preferred consistency

More water or ice can be added to help with your preferred texture/thickness.

26. Pineapple Protein Smoothie

Ingredients:
1 cup (135g) pineapple chunks
1 cup (200g) coconut milk (fresh or tinned)
½ med (65g) banana
¼ cup (65g) ice cubes
¼ tsp vanilla bean powder
pinch low sodium salt
1 tablespoon hemp protein powder

Instructions:
Peel pineapple and chop into small chunks.

Put everything into a high speed blender and blend until smooth.

27. Raspberry Coconut Smoothie

Ingredients:
½ - 1 cup coconut milk (depending on how thick you like it)
1 medium banana, peeled sliced and frozen
2 teaspoons coconut extract (optional)
1 cup frozen raspberries
1 tablespoon hemp protein powder

optional: shredded coconut flakes, and stevia to taste

Instructions:

Add coconut milk, frozen banana slices and coconut extract to your blender.

Pulse 1-2 minutes until smooth.

Add frozen raspberries and continue to pulse until smooth.

Pour into your serving glass, top with a couple of raspberries and a little shredded coconut, and enjoy!

28. Ginger Carrot Protein Smoothie

Ingredients:
3/4 cup carrot juice
1 tablespoon hemp protein powder
1 tablespoon hulled hemp seeds
1/2 apple
3 to 4 ice cubes
1/2 inch piece fresh ginger

Instructions:
Add to a blender and blend until smooth.

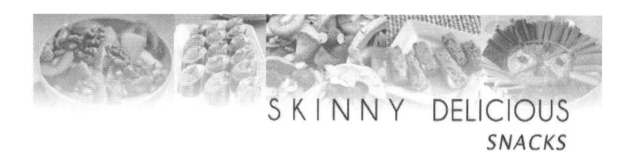

SKINNY DELICIOUS SNACKS

Paleo Epigenetic Snacks

1. Delish Banana Nut Muffins

Ingredients:
4 bananas, mashed with a fork (the more ripe, the better)
4 eggs
1/2 cup almond butter
2 tbsp coconut oil, melted
1 tsp vanilla
1/2 cup coconut flour
2 tsp cinnamon
1/2 tsp nutmeg
1 tsp baking powder
1 tsp baking soda
1/4 tsp low sodium salt

Instructions:

Preheat oven to 350 degrees F. Line a muffin tin with cups. In a large bowl, add bananas, eggs, almond butter, coconut oil, and vanilla. Using a hand blender, blend to combine.

Add in the coconut flour, cinnamon, nutmeg, baking powder, baking soda, and low sodium salt. Blend into the wet mixture, scraping down the sides with a spatula. Distribute the batter evenly into the lined muffin tins, filling each about two-thirds of the way full.

Bake for 20-25 minutes, until a toothpick comes out clean. Serve warm or store in the refrigerator in a resealable bag.

2. Delightful Cinnamon Apple Muffins

Ingredients:
1 cup unsweetened applesauce
4 eggs
1/4 cup coconut oil, melted
1 tsp vanilla
Stevia to taste
1/2 cup coconut flour
2 tsp cinnamon
1 tsp baking powder
1 tsp baking soda
1/4 tsp low sodium salt

Instructions:
Preheat oven to 350 degrees F. Line a muffin tin with liners. In a large bowl, add applesauce, eggs, coconut oil, stevia, and vanilla. Stir to combine.

Stir in the coconut flour, cinnamon, baking powder, baking soda, and low sodium salt. Distribute the batter evenly into the lined muffin tins, filling each about two-thirds of the way full.

Bake for 15-20 minutes, until a toothpick inserted into the center comes out clean. Serve warm or store in the refrigerator in a resealable bag.

3. Healthy Breakfast Bonanza Muffins

Ingredients:
8 eggs
1 cup diced broccoli
1 cup diced onion
1 cup diced mushrooms
low sodium salt and pepper, to taste
This recipe makes 8 muffins.

Instructions:
Preheat oven to 350 degrees F.

Dice all vegetables. You can add more or less of any of them, but keep the overall portion of vegetables the same for best results.

In a large mixing bowl, whisk together eggs, vegetables, low sodium salt, and pepper.

Pour mixture into a greased muffin pan, the mixture should evenly fill 8 muffin cups.

Bake 18-20 minutes, or until a toothpick inserted in the middle comes out clean.

Serve and enjoy! Leftovers can be saved in the refrigerator throughout the week.

4. Perfect Pumpkin Seeds

Ingredients:
1 cup of pumpkin (only seeds)
2 teaspoons of olive oil
1 tablespoon of chili powder (you may adjust it as per the taste you like)
1 teaspoon low sodium salt

Instructions:
Heat the pan (medium high heat) and place the pumpkin seeds.

After 3 to 5 minutes, you will hear the seeds making a crackling noise (some will even pop). You need to stir frequently.

Remove the pan and mix the seeds in olive oil, then low sodium salt and chili powder. Let it cool and then serve.

5. Gorgeous Spicy Nuts

Ingredients:
2/3 cup of each (almonds, pecans and walnuts)
1 teaspoon of chili powder
½ teaspoon of cumin
½ teaspoon of black
pepper (ground)
½ teaspoon low sodium salt
1 tables

Instructions:

Heat the pan on medium heat and place the nuts and toast them until lightly browned.

Prepare the spice mixture, while the nuts are toasting.

Mix cumin, chili, low sodium salt and black pepper in a bowl and add the nuts (after coating it with olive oil).

6. Krunchy Yummy Kale Chips

Ingredients:
1 bunch of kale, washed and dried
2 tbsp olive oil
low sodium salt to taste

Instructions:
Preheat oven to 300 degrees. Remove the center stems and either tear or cut up the leaves.

Toss the kale and olive oil together in a large bowl; sprinkle with low sodium salt. Spread on a baking sheet

Bake at 300 degrees for 15 minutes or until crisp.

7. Delicious Cinnamon Apple Chips

Ingredients:
1-2 apples
1 tsp cinnamon

Instructions:
Preheat oven to 200 degrees.

Using a sharp knife or mandolin, slice apples thinly. Discard seeds. Prepare a baking sheet with parchment paper and arrange apple slices on it without overlapping. Sprinkle cinnamon over apples.

Bake for approximately 1 hour, then flip. Continue baking for 1-2 hours, flipping occasionally, until the apple slices are no longer moist. Store in airtight container.

8. Gummy Citrus Snack

Ingredients:
3/4 cup lemon juice, freshly squeezed* and ¼ cup apple juice freshly squeezed
4 Tbsp. good quality vegetarian gelatin
liquid stevia to taste
1/4 tsp. ginger (freshly grated or ground)
1/4 tsp. turmeric (freshly grated or ground)

Instructions:
In a small saucepan, whisk together citrus juice, and gelatin until there are no lumps. Heat the liquid over low heat until liquid is warmed and gelatin is completely dissolved.

Remove from heat and stir in liquid stevia, ginger and turmeric with a spoon.

Pour into a casserole dish*.

Refrigerate until liquid is set (at least 30 minutes).

Serve cold or at room temperature.

9. Skinny Veggie Dip

Ingredients:
1 tblsp olive oil
1 tsp lemon juice
1 Tbs fresh minced parsley
1 Tbs french minced chives or scallion greens
1 tsp dried dill
1/8 tsp garlic powder
Pinch paprika
low sodium salt and pepper to taste

Instructions:
Combine in triple portions in blender and store to use any time.

10. Divine Butternut Chips

Ingredients:
1 medium butternut squash (400g / 14.1 oz)
2 tbsp extra virgin coconut oil
1 tsp gingerbread spice mix (~ ½ tsp cinnamon, pinch nutmeg, ginger, cloves and allspice)
pinch low sodium salt (or more in case you don't use stevia and prefer the chips salty)
optional: 3-6 drops liquid Stevia extract

Instructions:
Preheat the oven to 125 C / 250 F. Peel the butternut squash and slice thinly on a mandolin. If you are using a knife, make sure the slices are no more than 1/8 inch (1/4 cm) thin. Place in a bowl.

In a small bowl, mix melted coconut oil, gingerbread spice mix and stevia.

Pour the oil mixture over the butternut squash and mix well to allow it everywhere.

Arrange the slices close to each other on a baking tray lined with parchment paper or a rack or an oven chip tray (you will need at least 2 of them).

Place in the oven and cook for about 1.5 hour or until crispy (the exact time depends on how thick the chips are).

11. Outstanding Orange Skinny Snack

Ingredients:
1 T. vanilla extract
½ t. natural orange flavor
Pinch low sodium salt
1 ½ t. liquid stevia to taste
8 T. vegetarian gelatin
1 can coconut milk
1 ½ C. water

Instructions:

Heat water and coconut milk over low heat until simmering.

Continue on low heat, slowly adding in each tablespoon of gelatin, whisking the entire time.

Add remaining ingredients and whisk until any clumps of gelatin are gone.

Pour into molds, and pour remaining liquid into 8X8 glass pan.

Put in fridge until solid. …should pop out easily once hardened.

12. Spicy Pumpkin Seed Bonanza

Ingredients:
1 1/2 cups pumpkin seeds,
3 jalapeño peppers, sliced
3 tablespoons olive oil
low sodium salt and paprika, to taste

Instructions:
Preheat the oven to 350°F

Spread pumpkin seeds out on a rimmed baking sheet.

Add olive oil and low sodium salt and stir pumpkin seeds with your hands to combine.

Lay slices of jalapeño peppers on top of seeds.

Sprinkle paprika over the top of everything, generously.

Bake for 10 minutes.

Use a spatula to move the seeds and peppers around. Bake for another 5 minutes.

Move mixture around some more and bake for a final 5 minutes.

Remove tray from oven and let everything rest for 15-30 minutes to let the jalapeño-ness soak into the seeds.

Store in an airtight container...if you don't finish them all in one sitting.

13. Delectable Chocolate-Frosted Doughnuts

Ingredients:
For the doughnuts:
1 tbsp water, separated into
1/2 tablespoons
3 eggs
1 tsp vanilla
1/4 cup coconut flour
1/4 cup coconut oil, melted
1 tbsp cinnamon
1/4 tsp baking soda
low sodium salt to taste

For the frosting:
1/2 cup sugar free dairy free
Chocolate Chips
1 tbsp coconut oil

Instructions:
Turn on donut hole maker (You could also make these into regular donuts and cook at 350 for about 15 or so minutes).

Combine eggs, and vanilla in a food processor until well combined.

Add in the rest of the ingredients and continue to process until all ingredients are incorporated.

Add appropriate amount of batter to donut hole maker and use as instructed (Mine took about 3 or so minutes for each batch, but this will vary for different types).

While your donuts are baking, prepare the frosting by combing chocolate chips and coconut oil over LOW heat until melted.

Once donuts are completely cooled, dip each in frosting with a toothpick or skewer and completely cover, tapping off excess frosting. (I used a longer skewer stick and placed them standing up in a cup to harden, but if you aren't concerned with appearance, you can dip them with a fork or spoon, even, and just place them on a plate).

Place donuts in refrigerator to completely harden (about 1 hour).

14. Eggplant Divine

Ingredients:
1 large eggplant (about 1 pound)
1/2 cup olive oil
4 tablespoons balsamic vinegar
2 tablespoons pure liquid stevia
1/2 teaspoon paprika
low sodium salt

Instructions:

Wash eggplant and slice into thin strips. For ease in snacking you can cut long strips in half crosswise. Leave full-length for a more bacon-like appearance.

In a large bowl whisk together oil, vinegar, stevia, and paprika. Place strips in the mixture a few at a time, turning to make sure each is completely coated. If you run short of marinade, add a little more oil and stir it in with your hands.

Marinate 2 hours. Then, place strips on baking sheets

To dry in the oven: Line one or two rimmed baking sheets with parchment paper. Lay strips on sheets, close together but not overlapping. Sprinkle on a little low sodium salt (you don't need much).

Place in oven on lowest setting for 10 to 12 hours (ovens' lowest setting varies, thus drying time will vary) or until dry and fairly crisp, turning strips partway through. Check occasionally, and if any oil pools on the sheets, blot with a paper towel.

15. Choco Apple Nachos

Ingredients:
apples
fresh lemon juice
almond butter
chocolate chips
unsweetened shredded coconut
sliced almonds

Instructions:
Slice apples and toss with the lemon juice in a large bowl.

Arrange the apples in a plate and drizzle with almond butter. You can use a pastry/piping bag or a ziplock bag to drizzle the almond butter.

Sprinkle with shredded coconut, chocolate chips and sliced almonds.

16. Skinny Delicious Snack Bars

Ingredients:
1/2 cup almond butter
1 cup (250 grams) cooled roast pumpkin or pumpkin puree
3 cups desiccated coconut (finely shredded dried coconut)
1 (150 grams) ripe banana
1 teaspoon cinnamon
1 teaspoon vanilla
pinch of low sodium salt

Instructions:
Preheat your oven to 175 Degrees Celsius or 350 Degrees Fahrenheit.

Grease and line a 20cm x 20cm square cake tin with baking paper hanging over the sides for easy removal.

Place all ingredients into your blender or food processor in the order listed, blend to combine.

Press the mixture into the tin and cook for 30 minutes or until golden on top and an inserted skewer comes out cleanly.

Remove from the oven, leave in the tin for five minutes then carefully move the slice onto a cooling rack. Once it has cooled chop into bars. Enjoy!

17. Pumpkin Vanilla Delight

Ingredients:
115g (1/2 cup) pumpkin seeds
1 tsp vanilla extract
2 tsp liquid stevia
Water (boiled)

Instructions:
Preheat oven to 150c.

In a medium bowl, combine the liquid stevia, and vanilla. Stir together to create a thick paste then add a small drop of boiled water to thin it out and create a runny syrup.

Pour in the pumpkin seeds and stir them around in the mixture to evenly coat them.

Dollop a generous tsp full of the pumpkin seeds onto a baking sheet, repeat until it's all used up and cook for 15-20 minutes until most of the seeds have browned (but don't let them burn!)

Take out of the oven and leave to cool for a few minutes. Once they've cooled a little (but are still warm) you can press the clusters together to make sure they don't fall apart. They will dry quickly.

Once they're cooled and dried, they're ready to eat! Enjoy on their own or served on top of your cereal.

18. Skinny Quicky Crackers

Ingredients:
1 heaped cup of almond meal
1 egg
2 teaspoons olive oil
Pinch of low sodium salt

Instructions:

Preheat your oven to 180 degrees Celsius or 350 degrees Fahrenheit.

Place your ingredients into your blender or food processor in the order listed above, quickly combine at medium speed – you don't want the mixture to become sticky or turn to almond butter, although do not worry if this happens, it will still work.

Roll the mixture into a ball and place between two sheets of baking paper, roll out to your desired thickness.

Remove the top layer of baking paper and place on an oven tray. Bake for 20 minutes or until nicely golden. Remove from the oven and allow to cool prior to cutting into crackers. Enjoy.

19. Delectable Parsnip Chips

Ingredients:
500g (1.1 pounds) Parsnips
1/4 Cup Coconut Oil, Melted
3 Tablespoons liquid stevia

Instructions:

Preheat the oven to 200°C (392°F) and get out an oven proof dish.

Peel the parsnips and cut them into chip sized pieces and place into the oven proof dish.

Pour over the coconut oil and distribute evenly.

Drizzle over the liquid stevia and stir to combine well.

Place in the oven and cook for 15 minutes.

Remove from the oven and toss the parsnips over to allow the other side to brown.

Place back in the oven and cook for a further 10 to 15 minutes or until golden.

20. Spicy Crunchy Skinny Snack

Ingredients:
3/4 cup almond flour
1/4 cup coconut flour
1/4 cup flax seeds
1/4 cup of olive oil
1/2 tsp low sodium salt
1 1/2 tsp chilli
1/2 tsp cumin
1/2 tsp paprika powder
1 egg
1/2 tsp garlic powder

Instructions:
Melt the butter and basically mix up all the ingredients together, and knead it into a ball.

Take 2 sheets of baking paper, lay the ball on one, the other sheet on top and then flatten it out with a roller.

Cut triangles with a knife. Heat the oven to about 180C (350F) and bake for about 10 mins. Keep an eye on them so they don't burn.

21. Raw Hemp Kale Bars

Ingredients:
1/2 cup pistachios
1/2 cup pumpkin seeds
3/4 cup shredded coconut
1/4 cup orange juice
1/4 cup hemp seeds
1/4 cup coconut oil, melted
¼ cup dried kale crunched
3/4 cup dates, chopped

Instructions:

In a food processor, process the pistachios, pumpkin seeds, shredded coconut and dates until the mixture is crumbly but beginning to come together.

Remove to a medium mixing bowl and stir in orange juice, coconut oil, hemp seeds and kale.

Press into an 8-inch square cake pan or glass dish.

Chill in the refrigerator for at least an hour, then slice and serve.

22. Skinny Trail Mix

Ingredients:
1 cup flaked unsweetened coconut
1/2 cup raw almonds
1/2 cup raw pecans or walnuts
1/2 cup raw pumpkin seeds
1/2 cup raw sunflower seeds
1/2 cup dairy free sugar free Chocolate Chips

Instructions:
Combine all ingredients in a large mixing bowl and toss to combine.

Divide the trail mix between 9 sandwich baggies (about 1/2 cup of mix per bag) for a handy snack.

23. Anti-Aging Fruit Delights

Ingredients:
1 1/4 – 1/2 cups of pureed strawberries and raspberries
*If you prefer a less concentrated version, use 1 1/4 c fruit puree, and 1/4 c water!
4 – 5 tbsp vegetarian **gelatin**

Instructions:
Pureé the strawberries and raspberries.

In a small pan or pot on medium heat, whisk the gelatin into the fruit pureé until the gelatin is fully dissolved.

Pour the mixture into a glass pan. The smaller the size, the thicker the fruit snacks.

Chill the mixture for about 30 – 45 minutes in the fridge.

Cut into pieces and enjoy! Store in the fridge.

24. Paleo Rosemary Sweet Potato Crunches

Ingredients:
2 large sweet potatoes, peeled
1 Tbls coconut oil, melted
1 tsp low sodium salt
2 tsp dried rosemary

Instructions:
Heat oven to 375 degrees.

Slice sweet potatoes using a mandolin set to 1/8th inch.

Grind low sodium salt and rosemary with a mortar and pestle.

Toss sweet potatoes in a bowl with coconut oil and low sodium salt -seasoning mixture.

Place on a non-stick baking sheet (or a regular pan greased with coconut oil) and place into the oven.

After 10 minutes, take the pan out and flip the chips.

Place chips back in for another 10 minutes.

Pull the pan out and place any chips that are starting to brown on a cooling rack.

Place the chips back in for 3-5 minutes. Every oven is different so keep a close eye on the chips so they don't burn.

Place remaining chips on the cooling rack.

25. Apple Peach Skinny Bars

Ingredients:
6 Eggs
liquid stevia to taste
1 tbs (15 mL) Coconut Oil
1/2 tsp (2.5 mL) Vanilla Extract
1/3 cup (40 g) Coconut Flour
1/4 tsp (1.25 mL) Baking Soda, optional
1/4 tsp (1.25 mL) low sodium salt
2 tbs (30 mL) Applesauce
1/2 Peach, diced
1/2 Apple, diced
1/8 tsp (1 mL) Nutmeg
1/8 tsp (1 mL) Ginger
1/4 tsp (1.25 mL) Cinnamon

Instructions:
Preheat your oven to 325° F (163° C).
Grease an 8x8 inch pan (20x20 cm square) and line it with parchment paper.
Puree the eggs, liquid stevia, coconut oil, applesauce, and vanilla in a food processor or blender.
Add the coconut flour, baking soda, low sodium salt, and spices and blend until smooth.
Fold in the apple and peach
Pour the batter into the prepared pan and bake for 35-40 min or until a toothpick inserted into the center comes out clean.

26. Spicy Fried Almonds

Ingredients:
2 cups raw almonds, blanched*-boil for 3 minutes
2 tablespoons fresh rosemary, minced
2 teaspoons low sodium salt (or to taste, depending on how salty you like nuts)
coconut oil, or olive oil**

Instructions:
Heat a large pan over medium heat.

Add enough oil to generously coat the bottom of your pan (approx. 3-4 tablespoons), and allow to heat up.

Add the almonds to the pan. Stir frequently so that the almonds don't burn. The almonds will be ready when they're golden brown (approx. 5-7 minutes).

Turn down the heat to low and add the rosemary and low sodium salt. Stir well, and cook just until the rosemary becomes fragrant (approx. 2 minutes).

Remove the almonds from the pan and place on paper towel to drain any remaining oil.

Enjoy warm or once cooled.

27. Zucchini Avocado Hummus

Ingredients:
1 zucchini courgette, peeled and diced small
1/4 avocado (a generous tbsp's worth)
1 clove garlic
2 tsps lemon juice
1 tsp cumin
3 tsps tahini
1 tsp extra virgin olive oil

Instructions:
Stick all the ingredients into a blender and pulse until smooth.

Dust with paprika to serve and keep in the fridge for 4- 5 days.

28. Skinny Power Snack

Ingredients:
1/2 Avocado
1/2 tsp Paprika
1/2 tsp low sodium salt
1/2 tsp Garlic Powder

Instructions:
Sprinkle with all the seasonings and enjoy.

29. Skinny Salsa
Add any of the crunchy chip recipes mentioned in this book

Ingredients:
1 red onion, peeled and quartered
1/4 cup roasted hot New Mexico green chiles
6 large garlic cloves, still in skin
1/2 cup cilantro, chopped
1 qt cherry tomatoes
low sodium salt, to taste

Instructions:
Let the garlic roast for 5-7 minutes in a 200 degree oven. When the skins begin to darken, turn them over and continue to cook another 3 minutes.

Remove the garlic from the grill.

Now, place the tomatoes and onion in the grill Roast the veggies until nicely charred.

While the veggies are roasting, peel the garlic. Place the garlic in a food processor. When the veggies are finished roasting on the grill, add the tomatoes to the food processor along with the roasted New Mexico chiles and low sodium salt. Pulse to form a chunky puree. Pour into a mixing bowl.

Now, hand dice the onions and add the cilantro. Stir to incorporate and adjust seasoning, as necessary.

Pour into a serving vessel surrounded by your choice of skinny chips. Serve & enjoy.

30. Divine Turkey Stuffed Tomatoes

Ingredients:
2 lbs small tomatoes (bigger than cherry tomatoes, but small enough that you can eat them in two bites)
1 lb cooked turkey meat, chopped or shredded
2-3 stalks celery, finely chopped
3 Tbs minced red onion
1 carrot, peeled and shredded
low sodium salt and pepper to taste

Instructions:
Add the all ingredients other than the tomatoes and mix thoroughly. Taste and season with low sodium salt and pepper.

Cut a thin slice off the stem end of each tomato. Scoop out the insides (you can use your fingers but I used one of these scoops). Fill the tomatoes with turkey mix

Combine all ingredients. Refrigerate until serving.

31. Curried Nutty Delish

Ingredients:
2 Tablespoons organic curry powder
1 Tablespoon low sodium salt
liquid stevia to taste
2 Tablespoons water
1 Teaspoon olive oil
3 cups raw cashews, whole or pieces

Instructions:
Preheat the oven to 250F and line a baking sheet with parchment paper.

Mix together the first five ingredients and toss with the cashews.

Spread the nuts in an even layer and roast for 35-40 minutes.

Transfer to an airtight container. I made a bigger batch and put most of it in the freezer.

32. Skinny Chips

Ingredients:
1 (sweet potato) peeled and diced small
3 Small Parsnips peeled and diced small
4 lg cloves of garlic
1/2 Red Capsicum diced small
1 cup Flax meal
3 tbsp Chai seeds
1 tbsp Cumin seeds
1 tsp Smoked Paprika
1tsp low sodium salt
2 tbsp Olive Oil

Instructions:
Pre-heat oven 170c.

Place your raw diced sweet potato, parsnips, red capsicum, garlic and olive oil in your food processor and blend until into a fine mash.

Now that your raw vegetables are a mash add the rest of your ingredients. Blend in your food processor until well combined.

I then cut my dough into chip shapes with a knife on my oven tray. The key is to cut down rather that slice through.

I placed my ready cut "chips" in the oven. I pulled them out after 7 minutes and flipped them over.

After that every 3-4 minutes I turned them. I continued this over 20 minutes. (ovens will vary) I then turned my oven down to its lowest temp to dry them out further. This took a further 10 minutes. Remember each oven is different just ensure you have plenty of time during the cooking period to check and turn as needed. My oven isn't fan bake its old. So yours may crisp up faster!

33. Zesty Zucchini Pesto Roll-ups

Ingredients:
2 zucchinis
1 container of cherry tomatoes
1/2 c. pesto

For the Pesto:
1 c. fresh basil leaves
2 Tbsp. minced garlic
3/4 c. raw cashews
2 Tbsp. freshly squeezed lemon juice
1/3 c. olive oil
1 tsp. low sodium salt

Instructions:
Start off by making the pesto – mainly because it becomes more flavorful the longer it sits. Combine cashews, olive oil, basil, garlic, lemon juice, nutritional yeast, low sodium salt, and pepper in a food processor. Pulse until the consistency is mostly smooth. Cover and refrigerate.

Chop the ends off each zucchini. Then, using a mandolin or vegetable peeler, start peeling long strips from the zucchini. Repeat until you've peeled enough strips for the amount of rolls you want to make.

Have the cherry tomatoes ready in a bowl and a stockpile of toothpicks. On a flat surface, lay out a slice of zucchini, portion a spoonful on the strip and smooth it out evenly. Cover 1/2-3/4 of the strip, otherwise it will be hard to roll and the pesto will ooze out everywhere. Place a cherry tomato near one end of the zucchini and start to roll the strip around the tomato. When you get to the end, spear the roll with a toothpick and set it aside.

34. Butternut Squash-raw Veggie Dip

Ingredients:
1 cup cooked and peeled squash
½ cup COCONUT cream
½ teaspoon low sodium salt
1 teaspoon olive oil
1 ½ teaspoons finely chopped shallot
2 teaspoons fresh thyme
¼ teaspoon ground cinnamon
1 teaspoon chili powder

Instructions:
Place squash in a medium bowl and smash with a fork. Add remaining ingredients, mixing until thoroughly combined.

Serve dip with carrot sticks, veggies, or SKINNY CHIPS.

35. Skinny Power Balls

Ingredients:
1 medium size cooked sweet potato
2 cups almond meal
1 tsp vanilla powder
3 tsp baking powder
3 egg yolks
4 Tbsp melted Coconut Oil
liquid stevia to taste
3 Tbsp coconut flour (I used Coconut Secret brand)
1 cup of unsweetened shredded coconut and coconut flakes

Instructions:

Peel and mash cooked sweet potato until no more chunks left.

Mix in almond meal, vanilla powder, baking powder until everything incorporates.

Mix in the wet ingredients (egg yolks, melted coconut oil and liquid stevia), stir until everything combines.

Add 3 Tbsp coconut flour. Notice the mixture will be less wet but not too dry. Do not try to put too much coconut flour as it absorbs a lot of moisture and the balls would be too dry and flaky.

Line a baking sheet with a parchment paper. Pre-heat the oven for 350°F

Shape the balls into ping-pong ball size and roll each of them in the bowl of unsweetened shredded coconut and coconut flakes.

Bake the balls in 350°F for about 25 minutes or until the edges turned golden brown or they are dried out already. Remove from heat and let them cool down. The balls are soft when they're still warm but as they cooled down, they should be more firm. After they cooled down, put them in a fridge so they'll be more firm.

36. Chocolate Goji Skinny Bars

Ingredients:
1 cup raw cashews
1/2 cup cocoa powder
1/2 cup dried goji berries
1/2 cup hemp seeds
1 cup shredded coconut
2-3 tbsp coconut oil
liquid stevia to taste

Instructions:

Process cashews in a food processor until it turns into a paste. Roasted cashews don't work as well because they are less sticky.

Transfer paste into a large mixing bowl. Put coconut oil and liquid stevia into another smaller bowl and warm in the oven until it is fully melted.

While this is heating up, add the dried coconut, cocoa powder, and goji berries to the mixing bowl

Transfer melted coconut oil and liquid stevia into mixing bowl.

Everything should now be in the mixing bowl except for the hemp seeds. Mix everything in the bowl with a fork or your hands until thoroughly combined.

This should make a fairly mold-able dough. Spread the hemp seeds onto a plate. Begin to form your dough into small bite-sized balls and then roll them in the hemp seeds until they are thoroughly coated.

Pop in the fridge for at least 2 hours to harden them up a bit.

37. Delish Cashew Butter Treats

Ingredients:
1 Cup Cashews
Half cup coconut flour
0.5 Cup Cashew Butter

Instructions:
Add the cashews and cashew butter and process until the mixture forms a dough ball.

Add coconut flour to harden the mixture. You may need to scrape down the sides and help the mixture along to form a dough ball.

Once a dough ball has formed, move the dough to a plate to ensure there are no accidents with the food processor blade.

Form the mixture into 16 equal sized balls, refrigerate for at least an hour to harden and enjoy!

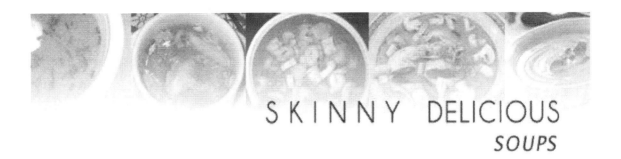

SKINNY DELICIOUS
SOUPS

Paleo Epigenetic Soups

1. Roasted Tasty Tomato Soup

Ingredients:
1 lb fresh tomatoes
1 red onion, medium
1 small head garlic, pealed
1 tbsp olive oil
1 tsp low sodium salt
1/2 tsp fresh cracked black pepper
1 tsp oregano
3/4 cup low sodium chicken broth, homemade preferably
15 oz tomato sauce, canned - sugar and salt free
chives to top

Instructions:
Preheat oven to 375 degrees F.

Cube tomatoes and onion. Place on baking sheet. Drizzle with olive oil and sprinkle with seasonings. Slice butter into small pieces on top of vegetables. Roast for 30 minutes, stirring halfway after 15 minutes.

Allow roasted vegetables to cool for 10 minutes. Purée vegetables, broth and tomato sauce in blender until smooth, scraping down the sides several times while blending.

Heat tomato soup in a sauce pan allowing the soup to slowly simmer for a few minutes to blend the flavors together. Serve hot topped with chives.

2. Thai Coconut Turkey Soup

Ingredients:
A small splash of oil
1 onion, sliced thin
A big handful of shiitake mushrooms, cut in half
3 cloves of garlic, finely minced
1 inch piece of ginger, julienned
A handful of cherry tomatoes
4 cups turkey stock 1 cup shredded cooked turkey (or chicken) meat
½ cup canned coconut milk
low sodium salt to taste
A small handful of cilantro

Instructions:

Stir fry onion, garlic, ginger and the add mushrooms and tomatoes.

Add turkey meat and fry for a few minutes till slightly browned.

Add stock and simmer for 20 minutes.

Serve warm and sprinkle chives on top.

3. Cheeky Chicken Soup

Ingredients:
2 large organic chicken breasts, skin removed and cut into ½ inch strips
1 28oz can of diced tomatoes
32 ounces low sodium organic chicken broth
1 sweet onion, diced
2 cups of shredded carrots
2 cups chopped celery
1 bunch of cilantro chopped fine
4 cloves of garlic, minced - I always use one of these
2 Tbs tomato paste
1 tsp chili powder
1 tsp cumin
low sodium salt & fresh cracked pepper to taste
olive oil
1-2 cups water

Instructions:
In a crockpot place a dash of olive oil and about ¼ cup chicken broth. Add onions, garlic, jalapeno, low sodium salt and pepper and cook until soft, adding more broth as needed.

Then add all of your remaining ingredients and enough water to fill to the top of your pot. Cover and let cook on low for about 2 hrs, adjusting low sodium salt & pepper as needed.

Once the chicken is fully cooked, you should be able to shred it very easily. I simply used the back of a wooden spoon and pressed the cooked chicken against the side of the pot.

Top with avocado slices and fresh cilantro. Enjoy!

4. Triple Squash Delight Soup

Ingredients:
1 butternut squash
1 gold acorn squash
1 white acorn squash
1-2 cups vegetable stock (depending on squash size, and how thick you want the soup)
2 cups diced turkey breast
1/4 cup light coconut milk
1 tbsp. olive oil
low sodium salt for seasoning

Instructions:
Preheat the oven to 400 degrees.

Halve each squash, scoop out the seeds (and saving them for toasting), and then slice into 1-1 1/2 inch thick crescents.

Spread the squash on an aluminum foil-lined baking sheet and coat lightly with the olive oil. Season with low sodium salt. Roast for about 30 minutes, or until golden brown (turning once mid-way through baking).

When the squash has cooled from the oven slightly, spoon off the meat from the skin.

In a medium to large pot, bring theturkey meat, the meat of all the squash and 1 1/2 cups of vegetable stock to a boil. Turn the heat to low and stir in the coconut milk.

Remove from heat to puree the soup. You can use an immersion blender, or transfer everything to a traditional blender.

Blend until smooth, adding any additional stock to achieve the consistency you like.

5. Ginger Carrot Delight Soup

Ingredients:
3 tbsp unsalted butter or coconut oil
1 1/2 pounds carrots (6-7 large carrots), sliced
2 cups chopped white or yellow onion
1 cup diced turkey breast
low sodium salt
2 teaspoons minced ginger
2 cups low sodium chicken stock
2 cups water
3 large strips of zest from an orange

Instructions:

Heat up the butter or coconut oil in a large soup pot.

Add the chopped carrots, turkey breast and onion to the pot and cook over medium heat for 5-10 minutes. Don't allow the carrots or onion to brown.

Add in the remaining ingredients (ginger, orange zest, water, and stock). The orange zest will be pulled out prior to puréeing so make sure they are in large, easy to identify strips rather than small pieces.

Bring to a boil then simmer for 10 minutes.

Remove orange zest strips.

Purée the mixture with an immersion blender. Or divide into 3-4 batches and blend in a regular blender.

I garnished my soup with a touch of olive oil and some freshly ground low sodium salt and pepper.

6. Wonderful Watercress Soup

Ingredients:
1 quart low sodium chicken stock
1 medium leek
1 bunch water cress
1 large onion
1/2 celeriac root skinned and chopped
2 cups diced chicken breast - organic
low sodium salt and pepper to taste

Instructions:
Gently heat the chicken stock in the pot.

In the fry pan sauté the onion, leek and celeriac until soft.

Place the onion, leek, chicken and celeriac in the pot of stock reserving 1/3 aside.

Season with low sodium salt and pepper.

Add the bunch of watercress and simmer a few minutes until it is wilted.

With the immersion blender blend the soup.

Add the chopped vegetables that you reserved, back into the pot.

7. Curried Butternut Soup

Ingredients:
2 medium butternut squash, cut in half lengthwise, seeds removed (save for garnish)
1 cup diced chicken breast – organic
1 medium yellow onion, chopped
1 inch piece fresh ginger, peeled and diced or grated
1 tablespoon curry powder
1 can coconut milk (find BPA-free coconut milk)
1 1/2 C chicken broth
Coconut Oil
low sodium salt and pepper

Instructions:
Preheat oven to 425 degrees.

Melt a tablespoon of coconut oil in a roasting pan.

Place squash, cut side down in roasting pan.

Roast 45 minutes to an hour, or until fork tender.

Add ginger and curry powder and saute 2 more minutes.

Scoop flesh out of roasted squash and add to apple mixture. Stir to incorporate flavors.

Add coconut milk, chicken and chicken broth. Stir to incorporate ingredients and bring to a boil.

Simmer mixture, uncovered for 20 minutes.

Using either a high power mixer or an immersion blender, blend soup until it's smooth.

8. Celery Cashew Cream Soup

Ingredients:
300 grams celery, washed and chopped
1 small onion, chopped
1.5 tbsp olive oil
500 mls vegetable stock
40 grams cashew nuts
low sodium salt and pepper to taste

Instructions:
Heat the olive oil in a large saucepan then add the celery and onion, stir to coat with oil. Turn the heat low and put the lid on leaving the vegetables to sweat for 5 minutes.

Add the garlic, give a quick stir then add the vegetable stock and simmer for 10 minutes.

Add the cashew nuts to the saucepan and simmer for another 5 minutes or until the celery is cooked through.

Tip the soup mix into a blender and purée until smooth.

Season with the low sodium salt and pepper and serve.

9. Mighty Andalusian Gazpacho

Ingredients:
3 pounds very ripe tomatoes, cored and cut into chunks
½ pound cucumber, peeled, seeded, and cut chunks
⅓ pound red onion, peeled and cut into chunks
⅓ pound green or red bell pepper, cored, seeded, and cut into chunks
2 cloves garlic, peeled and smashed
1½ teaspoons low sodium salt, plus more to taste
1 cup extra-virgin olive oil, plus more for serving
2 tablespoons sherry vinegar, plus more for serving
2 tablespoons finely minced chives
Freshly ground black pepper

Instructions:
Put all veggies in a large bowl and toss with low sodium salt. Let sit till the veggies have released a lot of their liquid.

Separate the veggies from the liquid, reserving the liquid. Place on a tray and place in the freezer for at least a half hour, or until they are partially frozen.

Remove from freezer and let thaw completely.

Combine the thawed veggies, reserved juice, oil and sherry vinegar in a large bowl. Ladle into a blender, working in batches if necessary, and blend on high until quite smooth. Chill for up to 24 hours.

Serve with extra sherry vinegar, olive oil and a sprinkle of chives

10. Munchy Mushroom Soup

Ingredients:
500g boneless chicken breast, sliced
150g button, straw or oyster mushrooms
1 large carrots, sliced
4 red tomatoes, quartered
6 cups low sodium chicken stock
2 stalk lemon grass, sliced into 1 cm pieces
juice from 4-6 limes (add more if you want it sour)
red chillies, chopped

Instructions:

Place the chicken stock in a pot, add lemon grass, and bring to boil over medium heat.

Add the chicken meat, mushrooms, tomatoes, lime juice bring to a boil and simmer for 15 minutes

Add sugar, chillies, carrots and simmer for additional 5 minutes.

Serve while hot.

11. Tempting Tomato Basil Soup

Ingredients:
4 cans whole tomatoes, crushed Note: check for ones without added sugar or salt!
4 cups tomato juice and part low sodium vegetable broth or chicken broth (I use 2 cups tomato juice and 2 cups low sodium chicken broth)
12 or 14 fresh basil leaves
1 cup coconut milk
Low sodium salt and cracked black pepper to taste

Instructions:
Combine tomatoes, juice and/or broth in stockpot. Simmer 30 minutes.

Purée, along with basil leaves, in small batches in a food processor, blender or better yet, a hand-held immersion blender right in the pot.

Return to pot and add coconut milk while stirring over low heat.

12. Healing Chicken/Turkey Vegetable Soup

Ingredients:
Coconut Oil 1 tablespoon
1 medium onion, medium dice
3 medium carrots, medium dice
1 zucchini, medium dice
¼ medium butternut squash, chopped into cubes
12 oz. container of mushrooms, rough dice
2-4 cups shredded chicken
1 tsp. dried thyme
1-2 tsp. dried rosemary + dried basil
½-1 tsp. ground cumin
1 Tbsp. Apple Cider Vinegar
Low sodium salt + pepper
chicken stock
Lemon {optional}

Instructions:
Get a big soup pot on the stove heating on medium with your favorite fat -- I liked coconut oil here because it really warmed up the soup's flavor!

Clean + chop your vegetables and add them in -- literally this is a chop + drop soup. Meaning as you chop just drop it all in and stir occasionally.

Add in as much chicken as you want, I did somewhere between 3-4 cups. I like a lot of chicken in my soup!

Add in your herbs, cumin, apple cider vinegar, low sodium salt + pepper and stir everything together well.

Add in your chicken stock -- I used around half of a batch but honestly just use as much as you want. You want it to cover the vegetables and chicken but after that it's totally up to you how much you add in. And if you don't have enough stock on hand you can always add in a little bit of water!

Stir everything up, cover {with the lid cracked just a little}, and let simmer on low for around an hour or until dinner!

When serving I like to squeeze on a little bit of fresh lemon juice! It makes it even more yummy that it already is!

Notes:
If you want to make this even heartier than it already is, you can add small layer of cauliflower rice to the bottom of your soup bowl, and then ladle the soup on top!

13. Sumptuous Saffron Turkey Cauliflower Soup

Ingredients:
2 tbsp extra virgin olive oil
1 medium onion, chopped (about 1 cup)
2 large garlic cloves, chopped
2 lbs frozen or fresh cauliflower florets
½ tsp low sodium salt
¼ tsp ground black pepper
5 cups of water or vegetable broth
20 saffron threads
Diced Turkey Breast

Instructions:

Sautée onion and garlic in olive oil on a soup pot, over medium heat, until onion is translucent, about 10 minutes.

Add cauliflower florets, low sodium salt and pepper and continue cooking for 10-12 minutes

Add 5 cups of water, bring to a boil and simmer until cauliflower is tender, 20-25 minutes.

Turn off heat. Add saffron, stir and cover. Let the saffron steep for about 20 minutes.

Blend soup in a blender until creamy.

Add Turkey Breast before or after blending

14. Delicious Masala Soup

Ingredients:
1-2 T coconut oil
1 large onion, chopped
2-4 carrots, chopped
3 garlic cloves, chopped
1 head of cauliflower, chopped up
3 cups low sodium chicken broth (or another broth you like)
Diced Turkey Breast
1 cup water
3 tsp dark mustard seeds
2 tsp cumin seeds
1 tsp ground coriander
1 teaspoon ground turmeric
1 tsp low sodium salt
1 T lemon juice
black pepper to taste
crushed red pepper to taste
Optional: chopped cilantro on top

Instructions:

Heat the coconut oil on medium-high and fry the onions, carrots and garlic cloves for about 5+ minutes until they are soft.

Throw in the cauliflower, mustard seeds, cumin, coriander and turmeric.

When the cauliflower is soft, add the chicken broth and water and simmer for 10-15 minutes.

Blend in the food processor until smooth (careful of the splashy hot lava liquid!).

Simmer for another 10 minutes (or until you're ready to eat), add the low sodium salt, pepper, lemon juice and crushed red pepper.

Top with fresh cilantro (I didn't have any, unfortunately) and add turkey breast and EAT.

15. Creamy Chicken Soup

Ingredients:
1/2 cup coconut oil, olive oil, or other oil of choice
2 stalks celery, finely diced
2 medium carrots, finely diced
6 cups low sodium chicken broth
1/2 cup cool water 1 teaspoon dried parsley
1/2 teaspoon dried thyme
1 bay leaf
2 teaspoons low sodium salt 3 cups cooked chicken, cubed
1 1/2 cups coconut milk (1 can full-fat canned or homemade; or pureed cauliflower; see Notes for alternate version)

Instructions:
Place oil in a large soup pot over medium heat. Add the celery and carrots. Cook, stirring occasionally, until soft, 10 to 15 minutes.

Add broth. If using arrowroot, place it and 1/2 cup cool water in a small bowl or jar and whisk or shake to combine. Add to pot along with parsley, thyme, bay leaf, and low sodium salt. Cook, stirring occasionally, until bubbly and thickened (if using arrowroot).

Reduce heat, just enough to maintain a boil, and cook, stirring occasionally for 15 minutes.

Stir in coconut milk (or pureed cauliflower) and chicken and heat through. This is a fairly thick soup; if you like it thinner, add more water, broth, or coconut milk and heat through. Remove bay leaf just before serving. Leftovers may be frozen.

Note:

Alternatively, you can use pureed cauliflower instead of the coconut milk. This version is just as creamy.

To puree the cauliflower, place florets from two medium heads in a pot. Optionally, add a peeled and smashed garlic clove. Add water to cover and about 1/2 tablespoon low sodium salt. Boil 20 minutes or until soft. Drain away water and puree until very smooth using hand blender or other method. Yield is about 4 cups; add the entire amount to the soup.

16. Delicious Lemon-Garlic Soup
Option – add 6 shrimps

Ingredients:
1 tablespoon olive oil
1 tablespoon crushed and chopped fresh garlic
6 cups good-quality low sodium shellfish stock (or mushroom or chicken stock)
2 eggs
1/3 to 1/2 cup fresh lemon juice
1 tablespoon coconut flour for thickening
1/4 teaspoon ground white pepper
chopped fresh cilantro or parsley, if desired

Instructions:
In a 4-quart pot, heat the olive oil over medium-high heat and saute the garlic for 1-2 minutes, or until just fragrant. Do not let the garlic brown.

Reserve 1/2 cup of the stock to mix with the eggs. Pour the remaining 5 1/2 cups of stock into the pot with the garlic. Let the mixture come to a simmer.

In a small bowl, whisk together the eggs, lemon juice, arrowroot, white pepper, and half of a cup of reserved stock. Pour the mixture into the simmering stock and stir until it all thickens--this will only take a few minutes.

Serve the soup hot, sprinkled with fresh cilantro or parsley.

17. Turkey Squash Soup

Ingredients:
1 large acorn squash
1/2 teaspoon olive oil
low sodium salt and pepper to taste
2 cups chicken or vegetable stock
1/4 cup coconut milk
1-2 turkey breasts shredded
3/4 teaspoon ground ginger
1 tablespoon coconut aminos
Pinch or two of cayenne pepper
Pomegranate seeds and/or sliced almonds, for serving

Instructions:
Preheat the oven to 400. Cut the acorn squash in half and scoop out the seeds and pulp. Brush each half with about 1/4 teaspoon olive oil and sprinkle with low sodium salt and pepper. Place in a foil-lined baking pan and roast, cut sides up, until fork tender (about an hour).

When the squash is cool enough to handle, scoop out the flesh and place it in a medium saucepan, or in a blender if you don't have an immersion blender. Add the remaining ingredients and process with an immersion blender (or regular blender) until smooth. Place the saucepan over medium heat and cook, stirring often, until heated through. Serve hot or warm, with pomegranate seeds and/or sliced almonds.

18. Roasted Winter Vegetable Turkey Soup

Ingredients:
2 large onions, cut into eighths
2 large sweet potatoes, peeled and cut into 1 inch dice
2 lbs of carrots, peeled and cut into 2 inch dice
1 head (yes head) of garlic, cloves peeled
4 tbsp coconut oil
low sodium salt and pepper to taste
2 cups low sodium chicken stock
1-2 turkey breasts

Instructions:
Preheat the oven to 425 degrees F.

Distribute the onions, garlic, sweet potatoes and carrots evenly on a sheet tray- it will likely require two trays.

Top the vegetables with coconut oil. You can melt the oil ahead of time if it is solid, or wait until it melts in the oven and then stir it around. Season GENEROUSLY with low sodium salt and pepper.

Roast for 25-35 minutes until vegetables are tender, flipping halfway through cooking.

When the veggies have roasted, transfer them into a large pot on the stove top. Add just enough chicken stock to cover the veggies by 1 inch.

Put the lid on and bring the liquid to a boil. Reduce the heat and simmer with the lid cracked for 10 minutes.

Now you get to puree your soup! You can do this in a blender, but do it in small batches so that it doesn't explode on you. But I love to use my immersion blender. It's convenient and you don't have to mess with all of the transferring and what not.

Taste and season with low sodium salt and pepper if needed.

Spoon it up and eat it as is, or stir in a bit of coconut cream add turkey- Enjoy!

19. Zucchini Fish Soup Delight!

Ingredients:
4 cups chicken broth , I used a low-sodium organic brand
2 cups zucchini noodles made with a spiralizer (2 zucchini)
2-3 cups cooked sliced white fish of choice
2/3 tsp fish sauce
1 1/2 tsp grated fresh ginger
Fresh herbs (handful): basil, mint, cilantro (whichever you prefer)
Sliced scallions, as much as you like
Thin slices of jalapeño
Lime wedges
Thin slices of red onion

Instructions:
In a medium-sized pot, heat the broth on medium heat until it becomes steamy.

Add the ginger (my favorite component!), , fish sauce and about 2 tablespoons of the herbs.

Simmer for a few minutes.

I added my jalapeño slices during this step because I like it spicier, but if you don't like it as spicy, wait until garnishing to add them.

Add your fish, zucchini and cook for about 4 minutes, until your noodles get soft and your meat is warmed.

Serve with the fresh herbs, jalapeño slices, lime wedges, and red onion slices as you like!

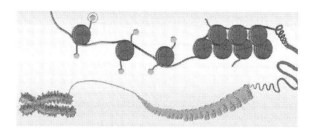

Chapter 11

The PKEVision

We've covered some very important ground so far in identifying the best ways to get you to the healthier, leaner, genetically smarter new you. Epigenetics prove in the clearest possible terms that we can influence and control our bodies at every level by taking control of what we eat and how we behave.

We've introduced you to the key points in your action plan for weight loss control and opened up a whole new world of health and wellbeing possibilities. But we have another important insight to share with you. And now is the perfect moment to reveal it!

Humans have a secret weapon in their behavioural armoury that can work powerfully to help us - or it can work just as powerfully against us. It's our imagination. Or rather it's our ability to visualise. Most of the time, our thoughts drift around in a random pattern of uncoordinated ideas, prompted by whatever happens to pop up around us. We are drawn to whatever grabs our fickle attention.

Our thoughts and feelings are largely conditioned from early childhood experiences that shape our future emotional framework. We learn from an early age to let our thoughts pretty much wander wherever they choose. The mind follows random currents, blown around like a leaf in the wind, lacking focus or any sense of direction. A ship without a rudder.

This is where the risks of self-sabotage emerge; uncontrolled thoughts and feelings, self-doubt, memories of failure, feelings of a lack of self-worth. The list is endless and potentially destructive to our plans for absolute wellbeing. So now is the perfect time to switch on our powers of visualisation and give the mind some clear directions to follow for the future. It's time to bring on the really powerful support system that is hidden within your own mind!

It's incredible to realise how much our expectations shape our perceptions and our behaviour. Our programmed attitudes and responses play a major role in determining many of the outcomes in our lives. Happily, humans possess the immensely powerful gift of visualisation.

By visualising a desired outcome, our behaviours shift to favour those clearly visualised results. The technique of visualisation is incredibly simple. All we have to do is relax. That's right. Relax. Sit down and relax and close your eyes. Now breathe a little more deeply. And see yourself exactly as you really, deeply desire yourself to be.

If you would like to learn more about the New Paleo PKE Diet, we suggest you download the initial book in this series at the following link

http://www.amazon.com/gp/product/B0131B2S5Y?ie=UTF8&camp=1789&creativeASIN=B0131B2S5Y&linkCode=xm2&tag=onelifeblog-20

Personal Vision - Summary

Engaging the power of visualisation

Meditating on the powerful new you

Building a clear picture of who you are becoming

Daring to dream and engaging the power of focused visualisation

Total health and well being

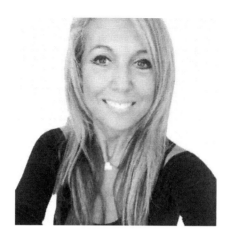

About the Author

As an International Nutrition and Weightloss Consultant, I have advised thousands of clients about successful weight loss strategies over the last 15 years

By the time I was twenty-two, more than thirty years ago, I began studying nutrition, integrative medicine and holistic health. I was immensely fortunate to find myself studying at one of the early pioneering centres of Integrative Alternative Medicine. This was the world renowned High Rustenberg Hydro, set in the beautiful countryside around Stellenbosch University, not far from my birthplace, Cape Town, in South Africa.

The Hydro at Stellenbosch, also known as the High Rustenberg Health Hydro, was founded by Sir Cleto Saporetti in 1972. The Hydro has become a world leader in holistic health and healing techniques, developing a range of methods to produce a balanced mind, healthy body and positive mental attitude. The original establishment comprised fourteen rooms and a staff of 25 under the supervision of Saporetti's co-visionary, Dr Boris Chaitow.

I studied very intensively for four years under the guidance of various medical and homeopathic doctors whilst also studying banking and finance. My studies continued right up until 1986 when I moved from South Africa to Europe.

The range of interests broadened, with certifications and examinations in Nutritional Therapy, encompassing naturopathic medicine, eating behaviours and disorders, orthomolecular medicine and the ancient Ayurvedic traditions that are witnessing a global revival after thousands of years of practise.

Those years of training, study, practise and experience are distilled and crystallised right here in your personal transformation workbook.

The reality is that I'm fitter and healthier today than at any other time in my life. Despite all the negative expectations surrounding the subjects of ageing and weight control, I can show you how to tame your body-fat problems and turn back the clock, helping you to find a younger, fitter, slimmer, stronger, healthier you. So let's get started!

Additional Books

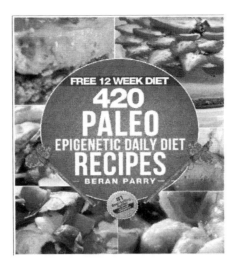

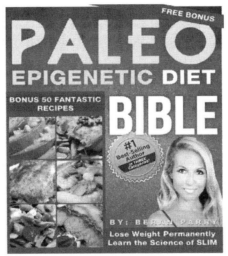

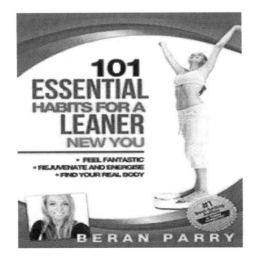

Bibliography

Scientific Studies General

Boling, C. L., E. C. Westman, W. S. Yancy Jr. "Carbohydrate-Restricted Diets for Obesity and Related Diseases: An Update." *Current Atherosclerosis Reports* 11.6 (2008): 462-9.

Cahill, G. F., Jr. "Fuel Metabolism in Starvation." *Annual Review of Nutrition* 26 (2006): 1-22.

Feinman, R. D., M. Makowske. "Metabolic Syndrome and Low-Carbohydrate Ketogenic Diets in the Medical School Biochemistry Curriculum." *Metabolic Syndrome and Related Disorders* 1.3 (2003): 189-197.

Liu, Y. M. "Medium-Chain Triglyceride (MCT) Ketogenic Therapy." *Epilepsia* 49.Suppl 8 (2008): 33-6.

Manninen, A. H. "Is a Calorie Really a Calorie, Metabolic Advantage of Low-Carbohydrate Diets." *Journal of the International Society of Sports Nutrition* 1.2 (2004): 21-6.

McClernon, F. J., et al "The Effects of Low-Carbohydrate Ketogenic Diet and a Low-Fat on Mood, hunger and Other Self Reported Symptoms." *Obesity* (Silver Spring) 15.1 (2007): 182-7.

Paoli, A., A. Rubini, J. S. Volek, K. A. Grimaldi. "Beyond Weight Loss: A Review of the Therapeutic Uses of Very-Low-Carbohydrate (Ketogethc) Diets." *European Journal of Clinical Nutrition* 67 (2013): 789-796.

Veech, R. L. "The Therapeutic Implications of Ketone Bodies: The Effects of Ketone Bodies in Pathological Conditions: Ketosis, Ketogenic Diet, Redox States, Insulin Resistance, and Mitochondrial Metabolism." *Prostaglandins, Leukotrienes and Essential Fatty Acids* 70.3 (2004): 309-19.

Veech, R. L., et al. "Ketone Bodies, Potential Therapeutic Uses." *IUBMB Life* 51 (2001): 241-7.

Volek, J. S., C. E. Forsythe. "The Case for Not Restricting Saturated Fat on a Low Carbohydrate Diet." *Nutrition and Metabolism 2* (2005) :21.

Volek, J. S., C. E. Forsythe. "Very-Low-Carbohydrates ." In *Essentials of Sports Nutrition and Supplements*, edited by Jose Antonio, Douglas Kalman, Jeffrey R. Stout, Mike Greenwood, Darryn S. Willoughby, and G. Gregory H., 581-604. Totowa, NJ: Humana Press, 2008.

Moore, Jimmy, and Dr. Eric Westman. *Cholesterol Clarity: What the HDL Is Wrong with My Numbers?* Las Vegas, NV: Victory Belt Publishing, 2013. Newport, Dr. Mary. *Alzheimer's Disease: What If There Was Cure? The Story of Ketones*. Laguna Beach, CA: Basic Health Publications, 2011.

Ottoboni, Dr. Fred, and Dr. Alice Ottoboni. *The Modern Nutritional Disease: and How to Prevent Them*, Second Edition. Femly, NV: Vincente Books, 2013.

Perlmutter, Dr. David. Grain Brain: *The Surprising Truth about Wheat, Carbs, and Sugar-Your Brain, Silent Killers*. New York: Little, Brown, 2013.

Phinney, Dr. Stephen, and Dr. Jeff Volek. *The Art and Science of Low Carbohydrate Living*, Beyond Obesity, 2011.

Phinney, Dr. Stephen, and Dr. Jeff Volek. *The Art and Science of Low Carbohydrate Performance*. Beyond Obesity, 2012.

Seyfried, Dr. Thomas. *Cancer as a Metabolic Disease: On the Origin, Management, and Prevention of Cancer*. Hoboken, NJ: John Wiley & Sons, 2012.

Skaldeman, Sten Sture. *The Low Carb High Fat Cookbook:100 Recipes to Lose Weight and Feel Great.* New York: Skyhorse Publishing, 2013.

Snyder, Dr. Deborah. *Keto Kid: Helping Your Child Succeed on the Ketogenic Diet.* New York: Demos Medical Publishing, 2006.

Taubes, Gary. *Good Calories, Bad Calories: Challenging the Conventional Wisdom on Diet, Weight Control, and Disease.* New York: Anchor Books, 2007.

Taubes, Gary. *Why We Get Fat: And What to Do About It.* New York: Anchor Books, 2011.

Tiecholz, Tina. *The Big Fat Surprise: Why Butte, Meat, and Cheese Belong in a Healthy Diet.* New York: Simon 8. Schuster, 2014.

Volek, Dr. Jeff and Adam Campbell. *Men's Health TNT Diet: The Explosive New Plan to Blast Fat, Build Muscle, and Get Healthy in 12 Weeks.* New York Rodale, 2008

Wahls, Dr. Terry, and Eve Adamson. *The Wahls Protocol: How I Beat Progreuive MS Using Paleo Principles and Functional Medicine.* New York: Penguin, 2014.

Westman, Dr. Eric. *A Low Carbohydrate, Ketogenic Diet Manual, No Sugar, No Starch Diet.* Dr. Eric Westman, 2013.

Westman, Dr. Eric, Dr. Stephen D. Phinney, and Dr. Jeff S. Volek. *The New Atkins for a New You.* New York: Fireside, 2010.

Keto Blogs and Websites

Everything About Keto, Reddit: www.reddit.com/r/

keto Ketogenic Diet Resource: www.ketogenic-diet-resource.com

The Charlie Foundation for Ketogenic Therapies: www.charliefoundation.org

Anderson, W. (2009) The Anderson Method: The Secret to Permanent Weight Loss. Minneapolis: Two Harbors Press.

Arem, R. (2012) The Protein Boost Diet. New York: Atria Books.

Baird, J. (2012) Obesity Genes and their Epigenetic Modifiers. Naperville IL: HWL, Inc.

Bouchard, C. (2010) Genes and Obesity, Volume 94 (Progress in Molecular Biology & Translational Science). Burlington MA: Academic Press- Elsevier Inc.

Campbell, T and Campbell, T.C. (2006) The China Study: The Most Comprehensive Study of Nutrition Ever Conducted And the Startling Implications for Diet, Weight Loss, and Long-term Health. Dallas, TX: BenBella Books.

Campbell-Mc-Bride, N. (2010) Gut and Psychology Syndrome: Natural Treatment for Autism, Dyspraxia, A.D.D., Dyslexia, A.D.H.D., Depression, Schizophrenia. Amazon Digital Services, Inc. [10 June 2014].

Carey, N. (2012) The Epigenetics Revolution: How Modern Biology is Rewriting Our Understanding of Genetics, Disease and Inheritance. London: Icon Books Ltd.

Chopra, D. (2013) What are you Hungry For?: The Chopra Solution to Permanent Weight Loss, Well-Being, and Lightness of Soul. New York: Harmony Books.

Cordain, P. (2011) The Paleo Diet Revsed Edition. New Jersey: John Wiley & Sons, Inc.

Dean, C. (2006) The Magnesium Miracle. New York: Ballantine Books; Updated Edition.

Ecker, S. (2014) Eating Well: How to build good eating habits to have your perfect body and overcome eating disorder. Available from: Amazon Digital Services, Inc. [2 September 2014].

Holick, M. (2011) The Vitamin D Solution: A 3-Step Strategy to Cure our Most Common Health Problems. New York: Hudson Street Press.

Kushner, L. et al. (2013) Practical Manual of Clinical Obesity. Chichester, West Sussex: John Wiley & Sons, Ltd.

Lask, B. (2011) Eating Disorders and the Brain. Oxford: Wiley-Blackwell.

Minger, D. (2014) Death by Food Pyramid: How Shoddy Science, Sketchy Politics, and Shady Special Interests Have Ruined Our Health…and How to Reclaim it! Malibu, CA: Primal Blueprint Publishing.

Power, M. and Schulkin, J. (2009) The Evolution of Obesity. Baltimore, MD: The Johns Hopkins University Press.

Sisson, M. (2013) The Primal Blueprint: Reprogram your genes for effortless weight loss, vibrant health, and boundless energy. Malibu, CA: Primal Nutrition, Inc.

Tollefsbol, T. (2014) Transgenerational Epigenetics. Waltham, MA: Academic Press- Elsevier Inc.

FREE BONUS CHAPTER

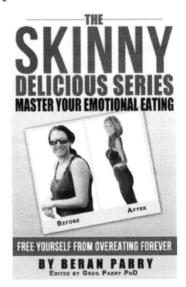

FROM THE MASTER YOUR EMOTIONAL EATING BOOK at

How Does EMOTIONAL EATING Really Work?

We need to start with a very important question. Are you ready for it? Here it is: "Why do we feel out of control?" The answers are very important to our understanding of how to introduce change to our eating habits. We feel out of control when we doubt themselves, when we feel frustrated, when we feel vulnerable or unsafe, when we feel rebellious or angry, when we feel empty, when we feel unexpressed and, finally, when we feel unfulfilled.

When a person crosses over the threshold between using food as a source of sustenance and food as a source of comfort, that is the moment when food easily becomes a psychological support instead of a biological necessity. Whilst we cannot always pinpoint why this might have happened, this book will help you to examine in depth your own unique responses in each of the categories and help you to be finally free of this pattern of unhealthy eating behaviour.

In the first part of the book, you'll be able to understand and interpret the insights to discover action you need to take to achieve real and enduring change.

Then, in part two, you'll learn about each of these fascinating steps and how they've been affecting specific areas of your life.

Together we'll remove each of the barriers and obstacles as you set sail on your personal emotional eating journey of discovery. And I'll be with you to help, encouraging and coaching you to free the real you that's been hiding for too long behind your emotionally-driven behaviour.

We'll look at why, after so many efforts to be free of uncontrolled eating, you're still at a place where you feel utterly lost. But don't worry. You'll certainly be able to begin again – this time with a renewed sense of expectation, realization and partnership. As you strip away each of the barriers, your emotional dependence on food will diminish until one day you will look back with wonder and ask yourself why you needed all that food in the first place!

Emotional Eating can be very well described via the following statements:

We eat to suppress our feelings of fear, guilt, resentment, worry, irritation etc.

We chose comfort food like cakes and biscuits and sweets because we felt we needed/deserved it and then felt guilty about it.

We ate badly to punish our bodies for some imagined failure in our lives.

This is a great moment to work through a simple quiz to determine whether you are in fact an emotional eater or someone who uses food to cope with the stresses of life.

Are You an Emotional Eater?

To find out if you're an emotional eater, answer the following five questions.

The last time you ate too much

1. When you needed to eat, did you feel a desperate and urgent need to eat something right away?

2. When you ate, did you enjoy the taste of every bite, or did you just stuff it in?

3. When you got hungry, did you need a certain type of food to satisfy yourself?

4. Did you feel guilty after you ate the same day or the next day?

5. Did you eat when you were emotionally upset or feeling that you "deserved" it

Let's see how you did.

1. Physical hunger begins slowly, then it becomes a stronger and finally it evolves into hunger pangs, but it's a slow process, very different from emotional hunger, which has a sense of urgency

2. There is a major difference between physical hunger and emotional hunger and it involves a degree of awareness. To satisfy physical hunger you normally make a deliberate choice about what you eat and you maintain awareness whilst you're eating. If you have emotional hunger, you won't notice how much you are eating or the taste and you will still want more food even after you're full.

3. Emotional hunger often demands very specific foods in order to be fulfilled. If you're physically hungry, even a salad will look delicious. If you're emotionally hungry, however, only your specific and possibly toxic choice will seem appealing.

4. Emotional eating often results in guilt. Physical hunger has no guilt attached to it because you know you ate in order to maintain energy.

5. Emotional hunger results from some emotional trigger. Physical hunger results from a biological need.

The Real Reason You're So Hungry – Imaginary Hunger

Did your answers to the five questions above reveal that you might be an emotional eater? Did you discover that you've been confusing emotional hunger with real, biological hunger? If so, the first question becomes – why?

The best way to explain what's going on is to consider that when you eat when you aren't really hungry, it's because you have two stomachs – one is real, the other imaginary. The hunger in your stomach is a signal to your brain that you need to re-fuel. It occurs when your system has a biological requirement for food. If that was the only signal of hunger you received, you'd be healthily slim. It's the imaginary stomach that causes the problems. The imaginary stomach sends out a signal demanding food as a result of complex and possibly negative emotions and unsolved problems. This is the moment when your stress and personal issues begin to assert themselves and you feel compelled to eat. Or, more accurately, to stuff yourself and anaesthetise the feelings of discomfort. Imaginary hunger exerts such a powerful influence that it compels you to eat almost anything to satisfy it.

There are certainly moments when each of doesn't really know what to do with ourselves. It can happen after work, when we are alone, late at night or even over the weekend. Does that sound familiar or do you have other triggers that compel you to sidle over to the fridge? All emotional eaters have specific issues that they want to avoid and, when those issues arise, the imaginary tummy howls with insistent urgency and you suddenly find yourself possessed by an out of control urge to eat.

SPECIAL FREE GIFT

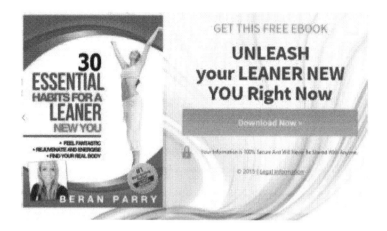

go to www.skinnydeliciouslife.com

BY THE SAME AUTHOR

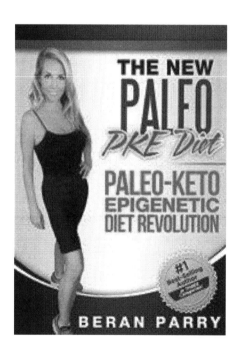

BY THE SAME AUTHOR

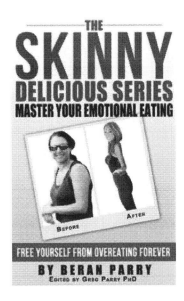

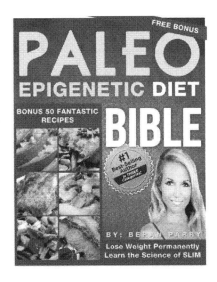

Made in the USA
Middletown, DE
16 May 2017